HOW TO
RECEIVE
AND
MAINTAIN
A
HEALING

Charles ✦ Fra

Published by
HUNTER BOOKS
201 McClellan Road
Kingwood, Texas 77339, U.S.A.

Books By The Happy Hunters

A Confession A Day Keeps The Devil Away
Angels On Assignment
Are You Tired?
Born Again! What Do You Mean?
How To Make The Word Come Alive
Follow Me
Go, Man, Go!
God's Answer To Fat...LOØSE IT!
Handbook For Healing
Hang Loose With Jesus
Heart To Heart Flip Chart
Hot Line To Heaven
How Do You Treat My Son Jesus?
How To Heal The Sick
How To Make Your Marriage Exciting
How To Pick A Perfect Husband...Or Wife
How To Receive And Maintain A Healing
How To Receive And Minister The Baptism With The Holy Spirit
If Charles And Frances Can Do It, YOU Can Do It, Too!
If You Really Love Me...
Impossible Miracles
Let This Mind Be In You
Memorizing Made Easy
Strength For Today
Supernatural Horizons
There Are Two Kinds Of...
The Two Sides Of A Coin
Why Should "I" Speak In Tongues?

In the event your Christian bookstore does not have any of the books written by Charles and Frances Hunter or published by Hunter Books, please write for a price list and order form from HUNTER BOOKS, 201 McClellan Road, Kingwood, Texas 77339-2710.

ISBN 1-878209-05-1

TABLE OF CONTENTS

For information about Charles and Frances Hunter's Evangelistic Census, Harvest Celebrations, and Healing Explosions, video and audio teaching and training tapes, books, or foreign languages for missions training, write to:

CHARLES ❤ FRANCES HUNTER
201 McClellan Road
Kingwood, Texas 77339, U.S.A.

On June 12, 1988, Cheryl Ingram, an outstanding psalmist and prophet, delivered a prophecy to our children, Bob and Joan Barker, concerning an attack that was going to come against us. This is what that prophecy said, in part:

"Satan has designed a very well-thought out, a very particular and a very detailed attack against Charles and Frances Hunter to discredit and invalidate their ministry.

Satan is even going to try to attack your mother's body!"

Foreword

One of the most unique, answerable, and yet unanswerable questions in the healing ministry is, "Why do some people get healed and others do not?"

And then to further complicate things, "Why is it that some people who get completely healed lose their healing?"

Is there more than meets the eye concerning not only receiving a healing, but keeping your healing and health once you have escaped from the hand of the devil! He is the culprit who dishes out sickness without regard to who you are, what your relationship to God is, the level of your faith, or anything else you could possibly think of.

This is something that has plagued many people.

Why is it that some people get healed and others do not?

Why is it that some great saint who has loved God her whole life and followed His direction, guidance, and Word, suddenly discovers that she is the victim of an incurable disease such as cancer, rheumatoid arthritis, or any one of the "impossible" situations which Satan loves to put upon us?

Why is it that this same great saint who has prayed for many people and seen them miraculously and instantly healed of all kinds of diseases, seems unable to receive a healing for herself.

Why is it that all the great "faith" healers can come, pray for her and seemingly nothing happens. Why is it this same great saint starts on a downhill path, dwindles down to absolutely nothing, and eventually goes on to be with God and Jesus after never being able to receive that special divine touch from God in her own life? These are questions all of us would like to have answered somehow or other.

We have made a lengthy study of this problem and while neither we, nor anyone else, have all the answers, we will give you some of the things which have helped us tremendously in receiving healings and maintaining them over the years.

We all know that the devil comes to steal, kill and destroy, and it is his plan and desire that those involved in the work of the kingdom of God will be the ones he attempts to "hit" the most. God's plan is that we live a long healthy life, so we need to know how to tap into that source of life and healing which will enable us not only to *receive* what God has for us, but which will enable us to *maintain* it!

Jesus is the giver of life and also the author and finisher of our faith, so we need to look to Him for the answers to those "unanswerable" questions.

One of the most critical factors in receiving and maintaining a healing, (because the answer in some cases is exactly the same), is to sincerely believe that God really wants to heal us. Some people hope, pray, think, wonder, question and doubt that God wants to heal them. Establish in your own mind and heart that God actually wants to heal you.

Probably one fact more than anything else has allowed me to be blessed and receive healing after healing and maintain them. That fact is this — whenever sickness hits, I know in my heart it is only a temporary thing, and I always know that I know that I know beyond a shadow of any doubt that I will recover.

This is not by "faith" or by quoting scripture, but is an honest statement of how I feel in my heart.

There is absolutely no doubt in my mind that God wants me healthy for the rest of my life because He has so much for me to do.

We hear so much about "incurable" or "terminal" diseases. The minute we hear that someone has cancer or some other "terminal" disease, we immediately panic and start planning their funeral. For some reason or other, doubt as to God's ability to heal them becomes an overwhelming thought and oppression that settles in on the majority of us. We try to push it aside, but it lingers there because the first thought that came into our mind said "fatal!" Pity, a tool of the devil, comes in because we feel so sorry for the person who has just received such devastating news.

Our immediate response to the news about someone's fatal illness should be, "I don't receive that in the name of Jesus!" and move in to attack!

God is never on the defensive, He's always on the offensive!

1 You're Dying...

By Frances

I have attempted over the last two years to try to establish when "it" started.

When was the first time I noticed there was something wrong?

Were there warning signals along the way that I ignored?

Did it suddenly sneak up on me?

Was there something I could or should have done to have prevented what the devil did?

I remember bouncing into the doctor's office for a quarterly check of my blood pressure and heart, feeling like a young sixteen-year-old girl. When the doctor asked me how I was, I said, "Fabulous — never felt better!"

His answer was quite a surprise and delight because he said, "It's always a pleasure to have you come into my office, because you always make *me* feel better!" Now that's a switch, isn't it, for YOU to make the doctor feel better? Charles and I both laughed because what the doctor really saw was our Jesus joy even though he is a Moslem from India.

He made the routine check and said all signs were normal, and then he said, "I want to take a potassium check on you." I willingly donated the little bit of blood required for that and Charles and I left home to minister healing out-of-town for about two weeks. I jokingly said, "If you find anything wrong with my blood, call my secretary, and she'll find me and deliver the news."

I knew there were no problems because I felt so good! Therefore it was shocking to receive a call from my secretary with the information that my doctor wanted me to start taking one potassium tablet per day and to come in to see him as soon as I returned home.

I purchased some potassium and took the one potassium pill per day, but it seemed to me I suddenly didn't feel as good as I had previously felt. I said to Charles, "I don't think those tablets agree with me," but because I believe when you go to a doctor you should follow his advice, I continued to take the one tablet per day.

As soon as we got home, we went right to the doctor's office for another blood test, knowing that everything would be fine!

I received a telephone call the next day saying, "Start taking two potassium tablets daily, because your system is extremely low on potassium." When you are not manufacturing sufficient potassium it can have a lot of side effects, some of which are not good at all. I mentioned to him that I had not seemed to feel as good after I started taking them as I previously had, and he said, "That's odd, because you should feel better."

I started taking two a day, confident I would be right back to my old vim, vigor and vitality which God has given me, but as I look back now, it seems to me I started on a slow, but definitely downward curve!

I suddenly noticed an unnatural "tiredness" which I would get, not on a regular basis, but enough to make me aware of it. Then it began to be more regular until one day Charles asked me if I was sure that the devil hadn't brought back diabetes? I insisted it was not a return of diabetes, because it was a "different" kind of tiredness.

We were scheduled to go to Japan, Taiwan, Red China and Hong Kong, so we went, positive in our hearts that this was a "temporary" thing and that I would be over "it" before we got to Japan.

I managed to make the two weeks' trip only by running to bed as fast as I could after each service or plane ride. It was a grueling trip, but it seemed to be much harder than any other trip had ever been on me. I said to Charles, "I guess I'm just getting older and can't do quite as much as I did before!"

The trip was finally completed, but we came back through Hawaii where we had another Healing Explosion scheduled! I remember when we got into the lobby of the hotel they told me our room wasn't ready, and it would be several hours.

I panicked! I was exhausted!

We called Bob and Joan's room, but they had

gone out, so I asked the management if they would let us in there because I could not sit up any more.

Complete exhaustion are the only words that express how I felt. It was such a tiredness that I felt my body wouldn't even sit up long enough to have our room ready. It got worse by the minute!

Before they gave the final okay to Bob and Joan's room, I was lying down on a couch in the lobby of the hotel! I wasn't worried what anyone would think — I was only concerned about the fact I never felt worse in my life!

I slept the whole day through, having allowed one day to recover before starting the Healing Explosion, and after sleeping that entire time, I got up exhausted! I managed to get through the first service (it's amazing what the anointing of God will do to give you strength!), but as soon as it was over, Charles literally carried me back to our room where I fell in bed exhausted. This continued throughout the entire Healing Explosion, even though I managed to make each service! I thought I was really suffering from "jet lag!"

We came home determined I was going to stay in bed until I fully recovered from "jet lag".

But that wasn't what happened!

The downward curve accelerated until it wasn't long before I discovered it was harder and harder to get out of bed in the morning and easier and easier to get back in early in the evening.

Then one morning I woke up and try as I would, I could not get up. As fast as I left the bed, I returned to it, fell into it and could not muster the necessary energy to stay on my feet.

I suggested to Charles that I might have caught the "flu" or something like that and that I was just "catching a healing" but that I would be all right by the next day. He prayed for me and went to work without me.

By this time the downward curve was diving almost straight down because daily I grew worse and worse. The office was praying, the church was praying, Bob and Joan's church was praying, but I still continued to get worse. We decided it was time to go to a doctor, so Charles literally drug me out of bed and we went to the doctor.

There was no fever, no nausea, no pain, only tremendous sweating, and extreme exhaustion. I could lay in bed wrapped in a terry cloth robe with towels on top of me, and in five minutes I would soak them all the way through. The doctor could not make a diagnosis, so he decided to make some blood tests. The first series of blood tests showed nothing, and I was getting worse and worse.

Then started a series of blood tests and tests of all kinds, and I proceeded to get worse and worse. I was tested for everything your blood can be tested for, and they all came out negative.

I'm sure the physician felt he had a hypochondriac on his hands, but I just didn't feel good, and yet nothing was showing up on any charts. He gave me some medication, including steroids (which I did not know about at the time) and all it did was make a tremendous weight gain!

Charles had to go on the road away from home

WITHOUT ME! On one trip I tried to go with him, got as far as Dallas, threw up all over the place, got violently ill, and he had to put me in a wheelchair, turn me over to the airline nurse, and run for his plane. One of the most difficult things in the world is to leave the one you love the most on this earth when they are sick. And the hardest thing for the one who is sick is to let their beloved go when you don't even know if you will live long enough to make it home on the plane. But one thing Charles Hunter and I know is that God has always come first, is always first in our lives, and will always come first in our lives regardless of the circumstances.

As Charles turned and waved at me, I could see him crying, torn between what he might want to do in the natural, but doing what he knew he had to do in the spirit! I couldn't even wave goodbye because my strength had gone!

Someone called my secretary, Barbara, to meet the plane with a wheelchair in Houston, and I managed to survive the 45 minute flight from Dallas, but when I fell in bed I was absolutely exhausted! She stayed all night at my house, watching over me like a mother hen.

I continued to get worse and worse. Even when you think you feel as bad as anyone can feel, you discover the next day you feel worse. It's difficult to understand how you can continually slide downhill when you have none of the usual things that indicate sickness, and I had none of them.

I didn't want to talk to anyone. I didn't want to see anyone. I didn't want to do anything. I didn't have enough strength to read the Bible, I didn't even have enough energy to think. It seemed as if I was in a bottomless pit with no way out, and even more devastating, no will to get out. I felt like a pile of nothingness lying in bed.

However, I didn't waste my time. My bed was stacked with piles and piles of cassette tapes. Pastor Gary Whetstone sent me about 150 of his tapes and I listened to his enthusiasm and anointing hour after hour which was feeding my soul.

I listened to tapes by Marilyn Hickey, John Osteen, and even my own! My body wasn't doing so well, but my spirit was soaring in spite of it!

I was too sick to read, too sick to sit up and watch video tapes, but at least I could lay in bed twenty-four hours a day listening to tapes. My sleep habits at that time were not good, so I went to sleep listening to tapes and would wake up while the same tape was still going. Even while I was asleep, I believe the Word of God was washing over me ministering to both my body and my soul.

There were many nights when my adrenalin was at such a high level because of being inspired by teaching on tape, that my heart would pound.

I would think, "Surely I can get up because my adrenalin is racing," but, try as I would, there was no strength in my body. Even getting to the bathroom which is just five feet from my side of the bed, was accomplished only by hanging onto the wall and the door!

The slide downhill seemed to be accelerating after my attempt to go with Charles, and at times it might have been easy to think that God wasn't going to heal me, but the only thing I ever thought was "When?"

Then one night something most unusual happened! I had apparently dozed off because I do not ever recall feeling as bad as I did that night. Suddenly — even though I was sleeping, — something roused me and I remember the horrible sickening feeling that engulfed me as the stench of death filled my bedroom. It was so horrible and so terrifying that I pulled the cover over my head in an attempt to escape whatever this was, and slipped back into apparent unconsciousness because whatever was happening was more than I could physically stand. I spoke the name of Jesus and slipped into oblivion.

I do not know what time it was when this was happening, but sometime after this I heard a telephone ringing in the distance. It was so faint I could hardly distinguish or recognize the fact that it was a telephone, even though it was next to my pillow.

I struggled to answer it, but I was trapped in something that I couldn't get out of, and that horrible stench was stronger than ever, and I knew I had to get out of whatever it was that was binding me. I continued to struggle to get out of what seemed like a huge pipe or tube, or possibly a tunnel which was holding me. It seemed like a hopeless task! After what seemed to me to be an endless struggle, I finally managed to get my head out.

The phone kept ringing and ringing, but I couldn't answer it.

I kept struggling and struggling, and finally

with supernatural effort, got my left arm out of the tunnel.

The phone continued ringing way in the distance! It seemed an eternity away! Somehow or other, I knew it was Charles calling me from somewhere, wherever he was.

With a divine energy, I finally picked up the telephone. He was still hanging on the other end, knowing I hadn't gone anyplace.

I did not say my usual greeting, "Hallelujah, God loves you," but weakly said, "Hello."

Charles apparently noticed something was seriously wrong with me and he said, "Honey, what's the matter?"

I replied, "I'm too sick to talk, please call me later," and with that I hung up and slid back into nothingness.

Hours later I woke up when my son-in-law Bob called me. Joan had just been operated on and was in the hospital and his loyalty was first to his wife, but his heart was breaking because he couldn't help me. Joan called me and all she could say was, "Mother, I wish I could be there to help you!" but she needed more help than I did.

I told Bob what had happened during the night, and with a love that very few mother's-in-law ever feel, Bob whispered, "Mother, did it ever dawn on you that you might have died last night and when Dad called you it brought you out of it?"

That had never entered my mind!

I said, "No way, I would have known it!"

He continued, "What time did it happen?" I

said, "Charles called me around 2 a.m. (4 a.m. Houston time) from California" because later I found out that the Holy Spirit had woke him up and told him to call me!

Bob continued with the greatest love imaginable and said, "That's the time of the night when your body is the weakest, and if Dad hadn't called, you might not be here this morning."

He promptly called our secretary and told her to stay with me until Charles came home. This is hard because she has a family, but praise God for her faithfulness and loyalty, she came over and "baby sat" with me until I felt I could once again be all right by myself during the night.

Bob and Joan called me three and four times daily to check on me and finally Joan was out of the hospital and Bob said, "Mother, we have such wonderful doctors up here, I think you should get up here somehow and let us take care of you. We'll make an appointment with some doctors to see if they can find out what your problem is."

In the meantime, Charles left for Sweden with a broken heart, but ministered with a tremendous anointing because we know that we know that we know that God has to come first, regardless of what the circumstances are!

How I got to Dallas was a miracle — it was a supernatural one — I could have never made it on my own! Bob met me with Joan lying down in the back seat, fresh from the hospital, so now he had TWO of us on his hands.

They had made some appointments for me, so

Bob took me to the doctor, left Joan in the car, but she couldn't stand not being with me, so she struggled up to the doctor's office, and what a day we had. I went from one doctor to another for a series of examinations and blood tests, blood cultures and everything else you could think of. When I related it to Charles on the telephone that night he said, "They were just trying to see what a faith healer is made up of!"

They decided there was a possibility I could have some disease I picked up in a foreign country. We had just returned from Japan, so they tested me for every "Japanese" disease I might have possibly caught. As I mentioned, we had come back by Hawaii and had a Healing Explosion there, so they decided it could be something from the South Sea Islands, so I was checked for everything they could think of from that area.

They even tested me for diseases that haven't been discovered yet!

I didn't have any of those diseases!

"Where were you before that?"

Brazil, Chile, Argentina, Paraguay and Uruguay."

Then I went through a battery of blood cultures for every disease known in those areas.

No diagnosis could be made!

Where do you go from there? Joan was exhausted, but they suggested a mammogram, so we went to a laboratory and had one made. No problems!

Where do you go next?

We all went home and went to bed, and Bob and Joan felt secure because I was in their tender, loving care. Charles felt peace since he could not be with me, because our children were taking care of me.

After consultations among themselves, the physicians decided I needed to see a specialist in Internal Medicine, so they made an appointment and off we went to see him.

Again I went through every kind of examination you can imagine — and then some. He decided on a series of blood cultures. I had blood drawn for seventeen, and for some reason or other, the blood was misplaced, and I had to go back and have it done again! Then we went through more series and more series of blood cultures. The beautiful, thorough, patient doctor to whom I went could find nothing, so I came back home to Houston because Charles was coming home.

I seemed to have reached a plateau of not going downward, not going upward, but at least holding my own, which wasn't very much, because I felt terrible. My strength was absolutely void, although my appetite was good, and I never had any fever, chills, pain, nausea, but felt terrible! Was this ever going to end?

Now let me back up a little! I am not telling you this story to give you the details of a horrible sickness, but to share with you some of the things I have learned on how to receive and maintain a healing!

Over the six-weeks period I was flat on my

back in bed, I received telephone calls every day from friends and well wishers who wanted to know how I felt. My answer was always the same: "Horrible" (and I wasn't being negative, I was just being honest), but each time I said, "BUT GOD'S GOT A MIRACLE AT THE END! Over and over I said those same words to person after person.

Many could not understand why I said I felt horrible. I said that because I was truthful, but watch what I was calling into being. A miracle from God! There was never a single moment when I had even one doubt as to the fact that God was going to heal me! I knew that I knew that I knew that this sickness was not unto death, but there was a miracle at the end.

I told many people that I didn't know what the miracle was, but I knew it was there.

I want to remind you of the words I said each time: "GOD'S GOT A MIRACLE AT THE END OF THIS!" Never one time did I give a report of my actual feeling without adding the miracle that needed to be called into being.

"GOD'S GOT A MIRACLE AT THE END OF THIS!" It wasn't just words that were coming out of my mouth. It was the heart-knowledge that I had of God's provision for me. I take seriously what it says in my Bible, "Frances Hunter, I wish above all things that you may prosper and be in health, even as your soul prospers!"

My soul was prospering because of the audio tapes I was listening to, so that is why I could confidently say, "God's got a miracle at the end of this!"

One day the telephone rang and the Internal Medicine specialist called me and said after discussing my case with many other specialists that they felt there was a possibility that I could have endocarditis, a fatal blood disease where the blood literally pulls off pieces of the heart until you die. He said I also could have a staphylococcus infection negative in the blood stream.

He said the treatment for this was hospitalization for thirty days, receiving massive doses of antibiotics twenty-four hours a day, and upon discharge the patient would have a shunt placed in the shoulder so that antibiotics could be fed into the body twice daily. I scribbled down all of these notes on a piece of paper by my bedside. *Then he casually mentioned that the disease was 100% fatal!*

All I could think of was that I didn't have time to go to a hospital for thirty days, because we had a Healing Explosion coming up which I had to attend! But then the thought came, "I couldn't possibly have something like that!" He said he would call me later as soon as the blood cultures had time to "cook" which takes seven days!

November 8, 1988 is a day I will never forget as long as I live.

I had not been to my office for six weeks, and it was election day. I did not feel good, but because Charles and I feel so strongly about Christians voting, we decided I should try to get dressed, go to the polling place, vote and then come home.

After we voted, I told Charles that I thought I could make it to the office so they would know I wasn't dying, because in spite of all this I didn't look sick! It was only when I got those awful spells of "sweating" that I was devastated. Sometimes they lasted for several hours! When I got over one, I was weak, but otherwise fine, until the next one unless I tried to get out of bed!

The staff was delighted to see I was still alive, but I had no more than walked into my office when the telephone rang.

Charles and I had prayed and prayed.

Many well-known Christians had prayed for me and nothing seemed to be effective!

Bob and Joan and Charles and I had prayed for every kind of disease and spirit we could think of but I still never was healed, but I always said, "As soon as we find out what this is, Charles will pray and I'll get healed!" We believe in specific prayers, and even though we know that God is sovereign and can do anything He wants to do and any way He wants to, we have found from much experience that it helps to know what the problem is.

I wasn't going to take the telephone call because I was sagging by this time, but when my secretary told me it was the internist, I grabbed the telephone. Our conversation is something I will never forget as long as I live!

Doctor: Mrs. Hunter, we have found out what your problem is.

Frances: Hallelujah! (Now I knew I could be healed because Charles would know how to pray!)

Doctor: You won't be saying that when you find out what your problem is... *You're dying!* (What a shock that was!)

I put my hand over the mouthpiece and said, "I don't receive that in the name of Jesus!" He was still talking!

Doctor: You have endocarditis, plus a staphylococcus infection negative in your blood stream! You have possibly six months maximum to live! I want you to be at the hospital tomorrow morning at eight o'clock. We will start you on massive doses of antibiotics immediately for thirty days. Then we will let you go home. We will insert a shunt in your shoulder and have a nurse come over daily as long as you live!

I personally believe your response at a time like this is critical as to whether you live or die. In the first place, *my spirit did not receive what he said.* I knew he was telling me what the laboratory reports said, but I knew what God was saying to me! Never was there one single moment when I believed I would die. I knew it was an impossible situation where I was concerned at that time. My mind raced, because I feel you should obey a doctor's instructions when you go to them.

What should I say to him?

What could I say to him? I had to go to San Antonio the next day to a Healing Explosion, and truthfully at that moment I don't know how I ever thought I could make it, but there was no question in my mind I would be there!

I said, "I can't. I have to go to San Antonio tomorrow. Can I come in Monday?"

He said, "No, I want you there tomorrow morning!"

I said, "I can't, could I make it Saturday?" thinking I could skip the Victory Breakfast! (By that time the Explosion would be over!)

Very sternly he said, "Mrs. Hunter, you don't understand! YOU'RE DYING! I want to prolong your life. I want to see you there tomorrow morning!"

MY SPIRIT NEVER HEARD A WORD HE SAID!

"I can't go to the hospital until I ask my husband if it's all right, then I'll call you back!"

The doctor realized I was making excuses and trying to wiggle my way out of going to the hospital, so as soon as he hung up, he called my daughter and said, "Please call your mother and tell her to be at the hospital tomorrow morning. She's dying, and she doesn't realize how sick she is!"

Joan said, "You don't know my mother!"

Praise God for a daughter who believes in the healing power of God!

Charles' office is at the opposite end of our building from mine, so I dialed him and told him the doctor had told me the problem and he came running down the hall, because now he knew that he knew that he knew I would be healed because now he would know how to pray!

I blurted out everything as soon as he came in sight of the door to my office. My words were coming out so fast, they must have sounded like a sentence without any spaces between words, "Thedoc-

torsaysI'mdying—thatI'vegotendocarditiswhichis
causingmybloodtopulloffpiecesofmyheart,anda
staphylococcusinfectionnegativeinmyblood-
streamandthatI'vegottobeatthehospitaltomor-
rowmorningateighto'clockandI"....

My husband, who loves me beyond measure,
didn't even say, "I'll miss you, honey." "What kind
of flowers would you like on your casket?" "I can't
live without you!" — not one of those things did he
say, and he never even let me finish my sentence, because Charles literally leaped over my desk, laid
hands on my heart and said, "In the name of JESUS
(the name where all miracles occur) I command a
total new blood system into your body!"

I felt nothing! No heat, no sensation whatsoever, but somehow I knew that my healing was
taking place. I merely said, "Thank you, Jesus!"

I dialed the heart specialist and told the nurse
what the internist had said and asked if I could see
the doctor immediately.

I don't care who you are, or how much you love
God, or how ready you are to go to heaven, receiving
a death sentence doesn't exactly turn you on! It
didn't turn me on either! They could sense the seri-
ousness in my voice and said, "If you can be here in
ten minutes — the doctor will see you."

Charles and I didn't say a word to anyone, but
dashed out of the office, jumped into the car and
drove as fast as we could up the highway! Charles
looked at me and said, "I've got peace!" I had just
told him I was dying and he tells me he has "peace"!
I knew that God had spoken to Charles to tell him

the situation was in His control.

I immediately began to put God in remembrance of His Word. I said, "*I shall not die, but live, and declare the works of the Lord* (Psalms 118:17). Then I said, "Father, you promised to satisfy me with long life and I'm not satisfied yet!"

I remember what I said over and over as I laid in bed,

> "*The Lord is my shepherd;*
> *I shall not want.*
> *He makes me to lie down in green pastures;*
> *He leads me beside the still waters,*
> *He restores my soul;*
> *He leads me in the paths of righteousness*
> *For His Name's sake.*
> *Yea, though I walk THROUGH the valley of*
> *the shadow of death,*
> *I will fear no evil; For you are with me...*"
>
> (Psalms 23:1-4).

God didn't say we'd sit down in the valley of the shadow of death, He said we would walk THROUGH it. Sometimes our steps may be weak and faltering and we may sometimes wonder if we'll make it, but if we will keep our eyes on Him, we will walk THROUGH any situation in life and come out on the other side totally VICTORIOUS!

Then another thought came into my mind. God had stationed a huge warrior angel with us in Abilene, Texas on February 4, 1978, and His words were forever burned into my heart when He said, "That's a special warrior angel I have stationed with you and Charles to protect you from the fiery darts of the devil until Jesus Christ comes back again! "

All of us have anchor points in our life. To some it is the day of their salvation — to others it can be almost any supernatural event in their life, but one of the anchor points in my life is that day when a big angel stood beside me and I heard the voice of God as clearly as I can hear my own voice!

I reminded God of what He had told me that wonderful, exciting day in Abilene.

All the way up to the doctor (which is only a ten minute drive from our office), I spoke scriptures concerning healing. Even though you can have the greatest faith in the world, a death sentence is still a shock to your nervous system, and to your "faith system"! I still wasn't turned on!

The doctor took me immediately, called the internist, and things really flew around the office. He told me to go to the hospital immediately for six more blood cultures because all of the more than one hundred previous ones had come out positive!

We went to the hospital and somehow when they took my blood, I knew this time it would come out right! The peace of God which surpasses all understanding had flooded my soul!

We left the hospital and immediately went to a Mexican restaurant and ate fajitas for supper! I will have to admit that there wasn't much conversation over the dinner table that night. Both of us were emotionally exhausted from the afternoon, so as quickly as we had eaten, we came home and immediately went to bed and fell asleep!

It was a GOOD sleep! The first good one I had

experienced in a long time and I was so grateful that I had fallen right to sleep without having time to stay awake or keep myself awake thinking about what had transpired during the day!

Somewhere in the middle of the night I was awakened. Either it was a vision or a dream, I am not sure which, because what woke me was a sensation that something huge had hit me on the head. It seemed as if it was a 2x4 piece of lumber, but our bedroom doesn't have that kind of a ceiling. As I mentioned, I am not sure if it was a vision or dream, but whatever hit me on the head bounced down onto my chest and when I saw it, it appeared to me to be a huge book which was open, and all I saw was one sentence, directly from God's Word:

"They that wait upon the Lord shall renew their strength; they shall mount up with wings as eagles; they shall run, and not be weary; and they shall walk, and not faint" (Isaiah 40:31 KJV).

I knew that I knew that I knew that God had healed me. It was a confirmation directly from the throne room of God, so I said, "Thank you, Jesus!", rolled over and went right back to sleep!

The next morning I woke up bright and early, feeling like a million dollars. Charles and I packed our luggage to go to San Antonio for the Healing Explosion, put it in the car, and then went to the "Infectious Disease Specialist" to whom the doctor had told us to go, but believing that we would go on to San Antonio.

He examined me, asked me an hour's worth of doctor-kind of questions, and I was bubbling over giving him the answers, when he said, *"What you did have you don't have! Go to San Antonio."*

We caught the plane and went to San Antonio, where I shared my testimony that night, and what a glorious Explosion we had!

We came home about a week later and my mail brought some interesting documents! It was the six blood culture results from the hospital taken the day I was advised I was dying! They should have gone to the doctor, but they came to me instead!

They came back negative, negative, negative, negative, negative, negative!

They asked me to come back and have six more made, because surely the blood had been mixed up! I did!

NEGATIVE, NEGATIVE, NEGATIVE, NEGATIVE, NEGATIVE, NEGATIVE!

Something had to be wrong! This never happens to blood when a person is not on medication!

NEGATIVE, NEGATIVE, NEGATIVE, NEGATIVE, NEGATIVE, NEGATIVE!

I was on no medication of any kind, so no "pill" can claim the healing. The doctor finally closed my case noting that the cause of healing was unknown.

Blood cultures do not instantly change from positive to negative in the natural, but I know God put His divine finger into my contaminated blood system and made it completely whole.

The medical profession might not know why or how I was healed, but I do, because I know the One who healed me, and I GIVE HIM ALL THE

PRAISE AND THE GLORY!

And I thank Him every day!

Please do not think that my comments are against the medical profession, because I appreciate what they do. When prayer doesn't get the answer we need, we do not hesitate to go to a doctor, which we feel is wisdom. People may say it's a lack of faith, but we feel it's the thing to do. Prayer always comes first, but when we are unable to somehow or other muster faith, or whatever it takes, we go to a doctor, and we appreciate them. I could have perished for lack of knowledge!

I appreciate with all my heart the doctors who talked with me for hours trying to discover the problem, made test after test, blood culture after blood culture and then gave me the diagnosis. I believe he was a stepping stone that God used to lead us into the right way to pray.

We do not ever question the sovereignty of God. He could have healed me any time any way He wanted to, but I believe He chose the way He did for some reason which we may never know until we get to heaven, but for whatever reason it was, I give Him all the praise and all the glory because He is the one who did it!

By Charles

Shortly after that, we went to a Healing Explosion in California.

I was at the booktable when Dr. Jantzen approached me and said, "I must tell you something."

He is a Spirit-filled doctor who had attended six or more Healing Explosions and who had helped us on Doctors' panels. He has spent a lifetime in medical practice.

He said, "Charles, when we received your letter asking us to pray for Frances, my wife and I immediately entered into prayer. Shortly after that, I went to my study and was impressed to pray in the spirit for Frances. An urgency arose in my spirit, and while seriously praying in the spirit, God said, 'Frances is going to die!'

"I was shocked. I said, 'God, that can't be so! You told her when you stationed the angel with her and Charles that they would live until Jesus comes back. They have so much important work to do for You!'

"That certainly caused me to much more seriously pray for her!"

When Dr. Jantzen told me this, instantly my mind raced back to what Frances had told me after the healing took place. I have read several books about people who died and came back to life again. They always remarked about going through a tunnel, seeing a light at the other end, and then coming out into that light.

Frances had told me about the horrible stench of death in our bedroom while I was away from home, and about how I had called in the night. I recalled how I suddenly woke up, felt an urgency to call her immediately, and did so. This was very unusual because I knew that was a time she should be asleep, but we must always be alert to the voiceless voice of the Holy Spirit.

When we wrote the book ANGELS ON AS-SIGNMENT, I had asked Pastor Buck if he went through a tunnel when he went to heaven, and told him that when God took me up to heaven in 1968 (see the story in FOLLOW ME), that I did not go through such a tunnel.

He said, "Neither of us died!"

What I believe happened was that Frances actually did die, that God had caused Dr. Jantzen to intercede seriously in praying in the Spirit, and had caused me to awaken her from what we thought was a deep sleep, but which I believe was death.

"When He came in, He said to them, 'Why make this commotion and weep? The child is not dead, but sleeping.' And they laughed Him to scorn. But when He had put them all out, He took the father and the mother of the child, and those who were with Him, and entered where the child was lying. Then He took the child by the hand, and said to her, 'Talitha, cumi,' which is translated, 'Little girl, I say to you, arise.

"Immediately the girl arose and walked, for she was twelve years of age. And they were over-come with great amazement!" (Mark 5:39-42).

For those wonderful six weeks (wonderful be-cause of what God could do even with just me minis-tering) horrible (horrible because my human heart was breaking, held together only by the assurance of both of us that we were doing what God wanted us to do). I was speaking in many places in the United States, in Sweden, Venezuela, and Costa Rica. During those six weeks I had heard testimonies from five healing team members of raising the dead.

Was Frances number six?

2   The Miracles of Jesus

One of the most important things in receiving and maintaining a healing is to believe that Jesus Christ is the same yesterday, today and forever, and what He did yesterday, He will do today and will continue doing tomorrow!

Thirty-seven specific miracles are listed in the New Testament and to believe them with our head is not sufficient. Until God gives us revelation on them, they remain only information, and nothing more, but once we receive that rhema word from God, they really come alive.

We read and reread all of the 37 miracles in the New Testament over and and over again because we believe the more that we can get the miracles Jesus performed when He was walking on this earth in our spirits, the easier it will be for us to not only receive a healing, but to maintain the healing!

Maintaining a healing requires as much faith as receiving the healing in the first place. Some of the 37 miracles Jesus did do not concern healing, nevertheless, they are in the miracle category and we need to get them down into our spirit so we can believe that with God ALL things are possible!

As we look at these miracles of Jesus as recorded in the four gospels, we must realize that these are only a "sampling" of all that Jesus did. *"Many other signs therefore Jesus also performed in the presence of the disciples, which are not written in this book, but these have been written that you may believe that Jesus is the Christ, the Son of God, and that believing you may have life in His name"* (John 20:30 KJV).

Those which the Holy Spirit chose to reveal to us were carefully selected from the thousands of miracles which we know Jesus did, so that from a study of them we might learn all that we need to know to both follow Him in the doing of miracles, and when needed, follow the examples given so that we may receive miracles in our own lives.

Each miracle is a demonstration of Jesus overpowering some principle allowed into the human race through the fall of Adam. Demonstrated is the control over NATURE, SATAN, DISEASE, PAIN, and DEATH.

Then He sent back the Holy Spirit to us and because of this He has both commanded and given us the ability to exercise that same total control over all that was lost.

There are many things which we need to watch for as we read all of the thirty-seven miracles, which are in chronological order. We want to encourage you to read every scripture verse carefully and not just skim over them thinking you know what they say, because they will speak to you in a new and different way.

You will notice that many times there is a cry of desperation. I wondered for years why it was so easy for people in the third world countries to be healed and much more difficult in the United States.

Here we always have an "alternative". We have hospitalization, medicare, pills and "remedies", but that's not present overseas. Their only hope is Jesus and in their desperation it seems easy for them to be healed!

If we can believe Jesus and use our faith, it's amazing how many times we have seen people healed the instant they "put their faith in action".

As we go through these miracles, watch for these signs, and also the action which I believe SEALS the healing — and will maintain the healing — the HEART OF THANKSGIVING. Many times we have seen healing released as the person simply stated from their heart — "THANK YOU, JESUS!"

MIRACLE NO. 1:
(John 2:1-11)

The first miracle that Jesus ever did was when he turned the water into wine, which appears in one gospel only! I have never been able to understand why all the miracles didn't appear in all of the gospels, but it is interesting to note how many times some of them appear and how few others appear.

The very first one Jesus ever did does not appear in any place exept John.

1. *On the third day there was a wedding in Cana of Galilee, and the mother of Jesus was there.*
2. *Now both Jesus and His disciples were invited to the wedding.*
3. *And when they ran out of wine, the mother of Jesus said to Him, "They have no wine."*
4. *Jesus said to her, "Woman, what does your concern have to do with Me? My hour has not yet come."*
5. *His mother said to the servants, "Whatever He says to you, do it."*
6. *Now there were set there six waterpots of stone, according to the manner of purification of the Jews, containing twenty or thirty gallons apiece.*
7. *Jesus said to them, "Fill the waterpots with water." And they filled them up to the brim.*
8. *And He said to them, "Draw some out now, and take it to the master of the feast." And they took it.*
9. *When the master of the feast had tasted the water that was made wine, and did not know*

where it came from (but the servants who had drawn the water knew), the master of the feast called the bridegroom.
10. *And he said to him, "Every man at the beginning sets out the good wine, and when the guests have well drunk, then that which is inferior; but you have kept the good wine until now."*
11. *This beginning of signs Jesus did in Cana of Galilee, and manifested His glory; and His disciples believed in Him.*

The first miracle Jesus ever performed involved marriage, which was the first institution God made in the beginning of the earth when He created Adam and Eve, so it is interesting to note that Jesus' first miracle concerned marriage. The family is close to the heart of God and I believe this is one reason that the first miracle Jesus ever did pertained to the family. However, the most significant sentence I believe is where Mary said, *"Whatever He says to you, do it"* (John 2:5).

Those words apply to us in our 20th century living. It doesn't make any difference what Jesus tells us to do, we need to do it. Not to question Him, nor to be disturbed by what He asks, but to just do it, regardless of whether it even makes sense to us in the natural, we need to "do" it!

I believe in receiving and maintaining a healing that this is one of the most important things to remember. Whatever Jesus tells you to do whether it's in the healing, in the maintaining, or living a Christian life, we need to do it! We need to be blindly obedient to whatever He tells us to do be-

cause when we are in line with Him then we can expect to receive the very best He has to offer.

MIRACLE NO. 2:
(John 4:46-54)

The second miracle Jesus ever did occurred
very early in His Judean ministry. It's also interesting in this and other miracles that He "abundantly"
supplied; not barely. Another result: The disciples
believed.

This miracle indicates what belief can do, be-
cause it simply says, "So the man BELIEVED the
word that Jesus spoke to him, and he went his way."
He did not question Jesus. He simply took Him at
His word. He did not say, "Keep praying for me!"
He simply believed what Jesus had spoken to him.
Belief can make your miracle come to pass!

46. *So Jesus came again to Cana of Galilee where*
    He had made the water wine. And there was a
    certain nobleman whose son was sick at Caper-
    naum.
47. *When he heard that Jesus had come out of Judea*
    into Galilee, he went to Him and implored Him
    to come down and heal his son, for he was at the
    point of death.
48. *Then Jesus said to him, "Unless you people see*
    signs and wonders, you will by no means be-
    lieve."
49. *The nobleman said to Him, "Sir, come down be-*
    fore my child dies!"

50. *Jesus said to him, "Go your way; your son lives." So the man believed the word that Jesus spoke to him, and he went his way.*

51. *And as he was now going down, his servants met him and told him, saying, "Your son lives!"*

52. *Then he inquired of them the hour when he got better. And they said to him, "Yesterday at the seventh hour the fever left him."*

53. *So the father knew that it was at the same hour in which Jesus said to him, "Your son lives." And he himself believed, and his whole household.*

54. *This again is the second sign that Jesus did when He had come out of Judea into Galilee.*

It is interesting and unique to note that this second miracle occurred when Jesus came again to Cana, which was the same site of His first miracle.

In verse 48, Jesus was so frank when He said, *"Unless you people see signs and wonders, you will by no means believe."* Jesus understood that so many people follow signs and wonders when actually signs and wonders should be following us.

All of us who are parents can understand the sincerity and the desire of the father's heart and also the fear in his heart because his son was sick. Any of us who have ever had a sick child know we feel exactly the same way. Jesus saw that the man had faith (not just desire) and so the son was healed. Another result: They believed.

MIRACLE NO. 3:
(Luke 4:28-30)

The third miracle was narrated in one gospel only.

28. *Then all those in the synagogue, when they heard these things, were filled with wrath,*

29. *and rose up and thrust Him out of the city; and they led Him to the brow of the hill on which their city was built, that they might throw Him down over the cliff.*

30. *Then passing through the midst of them, He went His way.*

This is a totally different kind of miracle because it's a miracle of Jesus being able to go right through a crowd without anybody ever seeing Him. When He walked on the water He was demonstrating a totally different kind of miracle but when he walked through the crowd He obviously either became invisible or He caused blindness to come over their eyes.

I well remember how Charles and I were at a meeting many, many years ago. We had flown to a meeting in the Ozarks which had been very hard to reach and we'd had to take several planes that day. We were totally and completely exhausted and had to be back to speak at a banquet that night.

Kenneth Copeland ministered in the afternoon, and at the conclusion of his service, he called us up on the stage, ministered to us in prophecy and we fell under the power of God. All the audience saw us, and they were aware that we were there, but as we walked among the audience toward the elevator, it was like they looked through us, but didn't see us.

There were probably 1,500 people there, and we had said, "God, somehow or another let us get to our room without people seeing us, so we can take a nap and be fresh for tonight."

We walked right through the crowd, not one person said a word to us, not one person stopped us. We got on the elevator which was loaded with people and not one single person acted like they even saw that we were there.

Nothing is impossible with God if we can believe it.

I believe one of the reasons so many different kinds of miracles were done was that God wants to show us that absolutely nothing in any way, shape or form is impossible with Him.

MIRACLE NO. 4:
(Luke 5:1-11)

1. *Now so it was, as the multitude pressed about Him to hear the word of God, that He stood by the Lake of Gennesaret,*
2. *and saw two boats standing by the lake; but the fishermen had gone from them and were washing their nets.*
3. *Then He got into one of the boats, which was Simon's, and asked him to put out a little from the land. And He sat down and taught the multitudes from the boat.*
4. *Now when he had stopped speaking, he said to Simon, "Launch out into the deep and let down your nets for a catch."*
5. *But Simon answered and said to Him, "Master, we have toiled all night and caught nothing; nevertheless at Your word I will let down the net."*
6. *And when they had done this, they caught a great number of fish, and their net was breaking.*
7. *So they signaled to their partners in the other boat to come and help them. And they came and filled both the boats, so that they began to sink.*
8. *When Simon Peter saw it, he fell down at Jesus' knees, saying, "Depart from me, for I am a sinful man, O Lord!"*
9. *For he and all who were with him were astonished at the catch of fish which they had taken;*
10. *and so also were James and John, the sons of*

> *Zebedee, who were partners with Simon. And
> Jesus said to Simon, "Do not be afraid. From
> now on you will catch men."*
>
> 11. *So when they had brought their boats to land,
> they forsook all and followed Him.*

This is an unusual miracle totally different
from all the rest because to me, this is a miracle
which indicates God's provision for you in all
things. They had fished all night long and had gotten absolutely nothing and yet I love what Simon
said in verse 5, *"At your word I will let down the
net."*

This is a case of a man who was probably totally exhausted after fishing all night. I am sure
there was nothing he wanted to do less than to throw
his nets out once again (he was already cleaning
them) and have to haul them in because there is a lot
of hard work connected with hauling in a net from
the sea whether it has fish in it or not. But his complete obedience saying, *"At your word I will let
down the net"* is something all of us should remember when we read the Word of God or when we
have a rhema word from God — "at your word I will
do whatever you tell me to do." When we "instantly
obey" without questioning God or trying to find
another way to do it, or an excuse not to do it, God is
pleased and will keep on giving you more to do for
Him.

This is a wonderful instance of Jesus showing
you that we can be looking for prosperity or a job in
one place and absolutely be unable to find anything
that is the least bit successful. Yet when He comes

along and puts His hand on it, as you can see in this miracle, they caught so many fish from fishing in exactly the same place that it filled the boats and the boats began to sink.

God always has a provision for you and not only a provision, He has a more than all sufficiency provision for you if you will just act "at His word".

MIRACLE NO. 5:
(Mark 1:23-28 & Luke 4:33-37)

This is narrated in two of the gospels.

Mark 1:23-28:

23. *Now there was a man in their synagogue with an unclean spirit. And he cried out,*

24. *saying, "Let us alone! What have we to do with You, Jesus of Nazareth? Did You come to destroy us? I know who You are—the Holy One of God!"*

25. *But Jesus rebuked him, saying, "Be quiet, and come out of him!"*

26. *And when the unclean spirit had convulsed him and cried out with a loud voice, he came out of him.*

27. *Then they were all amazed, so that they questioned among themselves, saying, "What is this? What new doctrine is this? For with authority He commands even the unclean spirits, and they obey Him."*

28. *And immediately His fame spread throughout all the region around Galilee.*

It appears a second time in Luke.

Luke 4:33-37:

33. *Now in the synagogue there was a man who had a spirit of an unclean demon. And he cried out with a loud voice,*

34. *saying, "Let us alone! What have we to do with*

*You, Jesus of Nazareth? Did You come to de-
stroy us? I know You, who You are—the Holy
One of God!"*

35. *But Jesus rebuked him, saying, "Be quiet, and
come out of him!" And when the demon had
thrown him in their midst, it came out of him
and did not hurt him.*

36. *So they were all amazed and spoke among
themselves, saying, "What a word this is! For
with authority and power He commands the unclean spirits, and they come out."*

37. *And the report about Him went out into every
place in the surrounding region.*

It's almost exactly the same in both versions,
but I'm referring to both of them so you can see what
it's talking about.

One of the things that impresses me the most
with this particular miracle is that Jesus did not talk
to the devil all night long, he did not argue with the
unclean spirit, but He merely told him to come out of
him.

Jesus knew who He was, there was absolutely
no question in His mind as to who He was and therefore, the demons had to obey Him.

The people were dumbfounded when they saw
His authority and yet He has given that same authority to us when He says in John 14:12: *"Most assuredly, I say to you, he who believes in Me, the
works that I do he will do also; and greater works
than these he will do, because I go to My Father."*

We need to remember when we use the name of
Jesus and speak with authority that the spirit will

come out exactly as it did when Jesus spoke a word.

When a person commands a demonic spirit to come out of you if you are sick, receive their word and be set free, because many sicknesses are caused by demonic spirits.

Cancer is a marvelous example of a demonic spirit. Christians and sinners alike get attacked by this horrible demon — but there is an answer, and that is to have the demonic spirit cast out with the power that's in the name of Jesus!

Several years ago we were at a meeting and a mother asked me if I had ever known anyone who was healed of epilepsy.

A young man standing there said, "May I answer that question for Frances?" Then he continued and said, "She laid hands on me 9 years ago and cast out the spirit of epilepsy and I have never had a seizure since that time!"

Just make sure the person who lays hands on you knows the POWER that is in the name of Jesus when they speak to the demon.

No loud shouting, no endless fight with the devil. He has to bow at the name of JESUS!

MIRACLE NO. 6:
(Matthew 8:14-15; Mark 1:30-31; Luke 4:38-39)

Miracle number six is a very unique miracle because this is the first one that appears in three gospels with the same story.

Matthew 8:14-15:

14. *Now when Jesus had come into Peter's house, He saw his wife's mother lying sick with a fever.*
15. *And He touched her hand, and the fever left her. Then she arose and served them.*

Mark 1:30-31:

30. *But Simon's wife's mother lay sick with a fever, and they told Him about her at once.*
31. *So He came and took her by the hand and lifted her up, and immediately the fever left her. And she served them.*

Luke 4:38-39:

38. *Now He arose from the synagogue and entered Simon's house. But Simon's wife's mother was sick with a high fever, and they made request of Him concerning her.*
39. *So He stood over her and rebuked the fever, and it left her. And immediately she arose and served them.*

The thing that is so interesting about this is that three of the gospels chose to tell this particular story and yet you will notice that each one only tells a very short version of the story.

In each case it said He came in and touched her hand or He took her by the hand, and in the third one it said He just stood over her and rebuked the fever.

In two gospels you'll notice the word *"immediately"* is used. In Matthew it says as He touched her hand the fever left her, which also means immediately.

Many thoughts come into your mind when you see this simple miracle repeated in three different gospels. Was it because mothers-in-law are not always held in high esteem and respect today, and God thought it would be a good idea to put it in there to show how much Peter was concerned for his mother-in-law? I do not know the answer to this, it was just an interesting little thought that came into my mind.

Another thing I like about this story is that it's such a very simple story. There was so little told and so little action done; it was simply a gesture or a touch on Jesus' part that created the miracle. If we can believe this for the miracle in our own life, if we can believe that Jesus can still reach down and touch us today, that's all it takes — there's just that one little spark of faith necessary to make a miracle occur in your life.

MIRACLE NO. 7:
(Matthew 8:16-17; Mark 1:32-34; Luke 4:40-41)

Miracle number seven is the second miracle that appears in three gospels.

Matthew 8:16-17:

16. *When evening had come, they brought to Him many who were demon-possessed. And He cast out the spirits with a word, and healed all who were sick,*
17. *that it might be fulfilled which was spoken by Isaiah the prophet, saying: "He Himself took our infirmities And bore our sicknesses."*

Mark 1:32-34:

32. *Now at evening, when the sun had set, they brought to Him all who were sick and those who were demon-possessed.*
33. *And the whole city was gathered together at the door.*
34. *Then He healed many who were sick with various diseases, and cast out many demons; and He did not allow the demons to speak, because they knew Him.*

Luke 4:40-41:

40. *Now when the sun was setting, all those who had anyone sick with various diseases brought them to Him; and He laid His hands on every one of them and healed them.*
41. *And demons also came out of many, crying out and saying, "You are the Christ, the Son of God!" And He, rebuking them, did not allow*

them to speak, for they knew that He was the Christ.

The thing that is so interesting about this miracle is the fact that Jesus healed all that were sick. Two of the three gospels report that they brought unto Him all that were diseased and that were possessed with devils and He healed them all! Only Mark says "many."

The two of us have often "laid hands" on the sick in crowds of one or two thousand people. Jesus often had far more people than that and He did it alone. If you lay hands on five per minute, it takes over three hours to lay hands on a thousand. It is exciting, wonderful and thrilling to see people healed with one touch of the power of God, but extremely exhausting. Jesus ministered day after day. When crowds exceed that, we must find other ways to minister healing. Now we have trained healing teams doing the works of Jesus.

Jesus has not changed from that time to this and so His desire is to heal all just like He healed at that time.

Again, you'll notice the Bible is very sparse in descriptions of these miracles because Jesus did them so easily, and I believe that's the way he wants us to do them today.

Many times a person's illness is not healed simply because we try to complicate the gospel so much instead of leaving it simple, exactly the way it was 2,000 years ago.

Jesus wants to heal you today exactly the way He wanted to heal all of them who were diseased at that time. He wants to heal all who are sick today. It's such a simple process if we can just keep it simple.

Don't struggle, strain or sweat to receive your healing — just relax and keep your eyes on Him!

He made it simple, and he expects us to keep it simple!

MIRACLE NO. 8:
(Matthew 8:2-4; Mark 1:40-44; Luke 5:12-15)

Miracle number eight — healing the leper, is in three of the gospels.

Matthew 8:2-4:

2. *And behold, a leper came and worshiped Him, saying, "Lord, if You are willing, You can make me clean."*
3. *Then Jesus put out His hand and touched him, saying, "I am willing; be cleansed." And immediately his leprosy was cleansed.*
4. *And Jesus said to him, "See that you tell no one; but go your way, show yourself to the priest, and offer the gift that Moses commanded, as a testimony to them."*

Mark 1:40-44:

40. *Then a leper came to Him, imploring Him, kneeling down to Him and saying to Him, "If You are willing, You can make me clean."*
41. *And Jesus, moved with compassion, put out His hand and touched him, and said to him, "I am willing; be cleansed."*
42. *As soon as He had spoken, immediately the leprosy left him, and he was cleansed.*
43. *And He strictly warned him and sent him away at once.*
44. *And He said to him, "See that you say nothing to anyone; but go your way, show yourself to the priest, and offer for your cleansing those things*

which Moses commanded, as a testimony to them."

Luke 5:12-15:

12. *And it happened when He was in a certain city, that behold, a man who was full of leprosy saw Jesus; and he fell on his face and implored Him, saying, "Lord, if You are willing, You can make me clean."*

13. *Then He put out His hand and touched him, saying, "I am willing; be cleansed." And immediately the leprosy left him.*

14. *And He charged him to tell no one, "But go and show yourself to the priest, and make an offering for your cleansing, as a testimony to them, just as Moses commanded."*

15. *Then the report went around concerning Him all the more; and great multitudes came together to hear, and to be healed by Him of their infirmities.*

In either of the stories, and it doesn't make any difference which version of the Bible you read or in which chapter you read, the message is exactly the same — it is the will of Jesus to heal you.

It is the will of Jesus that you be whole and that you remain whole. One of the things I think is so important is that we remember what the leper did when he came down to Jesus: he worshiped Him. Before he asked Jesus to heal him, before he mentioned anything about the desire of his heart, he fell down and worshiped the one he knew had the power and the authority and the will to heal him.

Many times we are so involved or caught up in our own particular situations and with the emergency or the crisis of the moment and the healing needed that we forget to take time to worship Jesus before we ask Him for what we want.

Then after the leper had worshiped Him, he so very simply said in Luke 5:12: "*Lord, if You are willing, you can make me clean.*" And Jesus said, "*I am willing; be cleansed.*"

Actually I love this story better in The Living Bible. The leper said to Him, "*If you want to, you can heal me.*" *And Jesus said, "I want to, be healed." And instantly the leprosy disappears.* (Matthew 8:2-3 TLB).

I guess the reason this touches my heart so much (and I hope it touches yours) is that Jesus is saying, "From the bottom of my heart with all that I am, I want to heal you. I don't want to see you on a sick bed! I don't want you to remain on that sick bed! And I want you, once you get healed, to maintain that healing."

I want! I want! I want! Jesus' "want" is to make you happy. Jesus' "want" is to give you the very desires of your heart.

I have certainly had some health challenges in my life since I became a Christian. I suppose this one particular scripture has helped me more than any other simply because whenever I read it or whenever I am in a situation where I need a divine touch on my body, somehow or another I can see Jesus saying to me, "Frances Hunter, I *want* to heal you."

In my spirit when I see this, I see Jesus with His arms outstretched to me ready to envelop just one of the five billion people on this earth.

Sometimes we might think, why would He want to heal me? His desire is to heal each and every one of us. And that's why I can see His arms stretched out and saying, "Frances Hunter, I want to heal you."

Put your name in the place of mine and know without a doubt that Jesus really wants to heal you. You don't need to beg or plead with Him — He WANTS to heal you even more than you want to be healed.

Right now visualize Jesus holding His arms out to you, saying whatever your name is — "I want to heal you." That's His desire, that's your desire and that's my desire, too. So just know that He *wants* to heal you. It's not His will for you to be sick, so let's get well and bless Jesus because He wants to heal us.

MIRACLE NO. 9:
(Matthew 9:2-7; Mark 2:3-12; Luke 5:18-26)

The ninth miracle that Jesus did again appears in three gospels.

Matthew 9:2-7

2. *And behold, they brought to Him a paralytic lying on a bed. And Jesus, seeing their faith, said to the paralytic, "Son, be of good cheer; your sins are forgive you."*
3. *And at once some of the scribes said within themselves, "This Man blasphemes!"*
4. *But Jesus, knowing their thoughts, said, "Why do you think evil in your hearts?*
5. *"For which is easier, to say, 'Your sins are forgiven you,' or to say, 'Arise and walk'?*
6. *"But that you may know that the Son of Man has power on earth to forgive sins" — then He said to the paralytic, "Arise, take up your bed, and go to your house."*
7. *And he arose and departed to his house.*

Mark 2:3-12:

3. *Then they came to Him, bringing a paralytic who was carried by four men.*
4. *And when they could not come near Him because of the crowd, they uncovered the roof where He was. And when they had broken through, they let down the bed on which the paralytic was lying.*
5. *When Jesus saw their faith, He said to the paralytic, "Son, your sins are forgiven you."*

6. *But some of the scribes were sitting there and reasoning in their hearts,*

7. *"Why does this Man speak blasphemies like this? Who can forgive sins but God alone?"*

8. *And immediately, when Jesus perceived in His spirit that they reasoned thus within themselves, He said to them, "Why do you reason about these things in your hearts?*

9. *"Which is easier, to say to the paralytic, 'Your sins are forgiven you,' or to say, 'Arise, take up your bed and walk'?*

10. *"But that you may know that the Son of Man has power on earth to forgive sins" — He said to the paralytic,*

11. *"I say to you, arise, take up your bed, and go your way to your house."*

12. *And immediately he arose, took up the bed, and went out in the presence of them all, so that all were amazed and glorified God, saying, "We never saw anything like this!"*

Luke 5:18-26:

18. *Then behold, men brought on a bed a man who was paralyzed. And they sought to bring him in and lay him before Him.*

19. *And when they could not find how they might bring him in, because of the crowd, they went up on the housetop and let him down with his bed through the tiling into the midst before Jesus.*

20. *So when He saw their faith, He said to him, Man, your sins are forgiven you."*

21. *And the scribes and the Pharisees began to*

reason, saying, "Who is this who speaks blas-
phemies? Who can forgive sins but God alone?"

22. *But when Jesus perceived their thoughts, He*
    answered and said to them, "Why are you
    reasoning in your hearts?

23. *"Which is easier, to say, 'Your sins are forgiven*
    you,' or to say, 'Rise up and walk'?

24. *"But that you may know that the Son of Man*
    has power on earth to forgive sins"—He said to
    the man who was paralyzed, "I say to you, arise,
    take up your bed, and go to your house." Jesus
    had the man put his faith into action.

25. *Immediately he rose up before them, took up*
    what he had been lying on, and departed to his
    own house, glorifying God.

26. *And they were all amazed, and they glorified*
    God and were filled with fear, saying, "We have
    seen strange things today!"

This is an especially interesting miracle because of what it says in each of the different versions. In Matthew it says, *Jesus, seeing their faith.*
Jesus looked on the natural elements and saw the
faith that they had.

Sometimes we say we have faith and we really
don't, but in each of these gospels it says, *He saw*
their faith.

Over in Romans the fourth chapter, it says we
can call into being those things which be not as
though they were. Many times God has to "see" our
faith and not just our words to know that we believe
what we say.

Jesus "saw" the faith of these men and that's

why the man was healed of paralysis.

This reminded me of an incident that happened while we were in Tegucigalpa, Honduras, Central America at a great Healing Explosion. It was difficult if not impossible to get down on the soccer field, so I told the people in the audience, "If Charles and Frances can do it, you can do it too."

I said, "If you have a disease, if you have an illness right now, I want you to put your hand on yourself and say, 'In Jesus' name!' It's that simple! "If I laid hands on you, I would believe that you were going to be healed, because Jesus said that those who believe would lay hands upon the sick and they would recover."

Then I added, "If you will do the same thing, that scripture applies to you just as well as it does to me."

There was a woman in the stadium who had an extremely severe case of palsy. She was shaking so badly she could hardly stand up and certainly had difficulty holding her arms out, but she heard those words, "If Charles and Frances can do it, you can do it too!"

Faith ignited in her that she had never had before because she was not a saved person. But she believed, and I believe God *saw her faith* to believe that if she touched herself she would be healed! She laid hands on her forehead and said, "In Jesus' name, be healed." The palsy was instantly healed and she immediately stopped shaking.

She went back to the doctor to confirm her healing and he could find absolutely not one hangover from the palsy. As a result of this, she accepted Jesus as her Savior and Lord!

Healing is a tool God has given us so that the world will believe that Jesus is alive today.

I want you to really think about that and lay hands on yourself right now and say, "If that woman in Tegucigalpa can do it, I can do it too. If Jesus saw the faith of those men, let Him see my faith too."

Don't think you can "con" God or "con" Jesus, because you can't. I've heard so many people say, "Tonight is my night to be healed, tonight I know I'm going to be healed." And yet in my spirit, I know they don't have a single solitary bit of faith.

Don't let that happen to you. Get your "expectors" up, put your feet on the solid ground of the Word, and get your belief going in the right direction!

It works!

MIRACLE NO. 10:
(John 5:2-16)

The tenth miracle that Jesus did is narrated in one gospel only.

John 5:2-16

2. *Now there is in Jerusalem by the Sheep Gate a pool, which is called in Hebrew, Bethesda, having five porches.*
3. *In these lay a great multitude of sick people, blind, lame, paralyzed, waiting for the moving of the water.*
4. *For an angel went down at a certain time into the pool and stirred up the water; then whoever stepped in first, after the stirring of the water, was made well of whatever disease he had.*
5. *Now a certain man was there who had an infirmity thirty-eight years.*
6. *When Jesus saw him lying there, and knew that he already had been in that condition a long time, He said to him, "Do you want to be made well?"* Again, Jesus required faith to be put into action.
7. *The sick man answered Him, "Sir, I have no man to put me into the pool when the water is stirred up; but while I am coming, another steps down before me."*
8. *Jesus said to him, "Rise, take up your bed and walk."*

9. *And immediately the man was made well, took up his bed, and walked. And that day was the Sabbath.*

10. *The Jews therefore said to him who was cured, "It is the Sabbath; it is not lawful for you to carry your bed."*

11. *He answered them, "He who made me well said to me, 'Take up your bed and walk.'"*

12. *Then they asked him, "Who is the Man who said to you, 'Take up your bed and walk'?"*

13. *But the one who was healed did not know who it was, for Jesus had withdrawn, a multitude being in that place.*

14. *Afterward Jesus found him in the temple, and said to him, "See, you have been made well. Sin no more, lest a worse thing come upon you."*

15. *The man departed and told the Jews that it was Jesus who had made him well.*

16. *For this reason the Jews persecuted Jesus, and sought to kill Him, because He had done these things on the Sabbath.*

I think it's interesting to note, if you will, that most of the time when John related a miracle he was the only one who related that particular event. I have never been able to figure this out, but I think it's an unusual fact anyway. This is an interesting type of healing because it was a well-known fact that when the angel came down and troubled the water, the first one who got in after the troubling of the water was made whole regardless of what disease he had.

I'm sure that there is a purpose in this miracle

far greater than any of us can realize or certainly far greater than I can realize. The thing I'm wondering is this, was it only the first one who got in there who got healed because that first one really believed?

Is that why he got in there in such a hurry, or was it the fact that a lot of people once they "enjoy" a sickness never seem to mind suffering with that sickness?

A lot of people love to talk about their sicknesses and that's why I think it's hard sometimes for certain people to get healed. They hang on to illness like a security blanket.

Did you notice the question that Jesus asked the man in verse 6? He said, *"Do you want to be made well?"*

If you'll notice, the man did not say, "Yes." He just simply gave an excuse saying in verse 7, *"I have no man to put me in the pool when the water is stirred up."*

I think we need to establish in our mind that we absolutely *want* to be healed. Whether it's a big sickness or a little sickness we need to *want* to recover! Not only do we need to know that Jesus wants to heal us, we need to want to be healed ourself.

Now you might say that's a very odd kind of reasoning, everybody wants to be healed and yet, there are many times when I wonder if we don't just tolerate a sickness because we know its just a little temporary thing and we're going to get over it very quickly.

Did you ever start to get a cold and then say,

"Oh, well, I'll be over this in a few days." Really saying, "I don't want to be healed, I know that I'll get over this in just a few days so I don't really have to be healed." That's a very interesting type of reasoning and I just wanted to put that in your mind because I think that was the problem the man had all the time. He kept looking at excuses rather than at being healed.

Some people enjoy the attention they receive while they are sick. That's detrimental to healing!

Look for the healing and not for the excuse!

MIRACLE NO. 11:
(Matthew 12:10-13; Mark 3:1-5; Luke 6:6-10)

Miracle number eleven is found in three gospels. The fact I have found interesting in making this study is that when it appears in three, it appears in Matthew, Mark and Luke. The single ones appear mostly in the book of John. Maybe that's because three of them were similar and the fourth one, John, was different than the rest. I don't know, that's just a thought that I throw out to you.

Matthew 12:10-13:

10. *And behold, there was a man who had a withered hand. And they asked Him, saying, "Is it lawful to heal on the Sabbath?" — that they might accuse Him.*
11. *Then He said to them, "What man is there among you who has one sheep, and if it falls into a pit on the Sabbath, will not lay hold of it and lift it out?*
12. *Of how much more value then is a man than a sheep? Therefore it is lawful to do good on the Sabbath."*
13. *Then He said to the man, "Stretch out your hand." And he stretched it out, and it was restored as whole as the other.*

I think this miracle is especially fascinating because it concerns a man with a withered hand and the first question that was asked Jesus was by the skeptics, the unbelievers, and those who liked to antagonize Christians! Look at the legalistic question in Verse 10: *"Is it lawful to heal on the Sabbath?"*

We face exactly the same thing today. "Do you really think it's God's will to heal everyone?" "Does God put sickness upon us to teach us a lesson?" Answering the first question, "Yes, God does want you healed; second, God does not put sickness upon you to teach you a lesson." (Matthew 8:1-5).

These are questions often asked of us and many more in a similar vein simply through legalism and a lack of faith and a lack of believing that God really wants to heal people.

If you'll notice they started this off with a question of unbelief and doubt and a sincere desire to see that the man was not healed.

I love it when Jesus just said, Verse 12: *"Of how much more value is a man than a sheep? Therefore it is lawful to do good on the Sabbath."* Jesus told the man, *"Stretch out your hand"* and the man was instantly healed, overriding all the legalism that was there.

Mark 3:1-5:

1. *And He entered the synagogue again, and a man was there who had a withered hand.*
2. *And they watched Him closely, whether He would heal him on the Sabbath, so that they might accuse Him.*
3. *Then He said to the man who had the withered hand, "Step forward."*
4. *And He said to them, "Is it lawful on the Sabbath to do good or to do evil, to save life or to kill?" But they kept silent.*

5. *So when He had looked around at them with anger, being grieved by the hardness of their hearts, He said to the man, "Stretch out your hand." And he stretched it out, and his hand was restored as whole as the other.*

Luke 6:6-10:

6. *Now it happened on another Sabbath, also, that He entered the synagogue and taught. And a man was there whose right hand was withered.*
7. *And the scribes and Pharisees watched Him closely, whether He would heal on the Sabbath, that they might find an accusation against Him.*
8. *But He knew their thoughts, and said to the man who had the withered hand, "Arise and stand here." And he arose and stood.*
9. *Then Jesus said to them, "I will ask you one thing: Is it lawful on the Sabbath to do good or to do evil, to save life or to destroy it?"*
10. *And looking around at them all, He said to the man, "Stretch out your hand." And he did so, and his hand was restored as whole as the other.*

Many times the stories as they appear in the different gospels are almost identical and yet if you will read each one you'll notice there's something that's a little different. In the book of Luke, verse 8 it said, *"He knew their thoughts."* He knew that the legalistic Pharisees were trying to find some kind of accusation against Him, but again, the end result was exactly the same — the man was healed. Beware of legalism and don't back down!

MIRACLE NO. 12:
(Matthew 8:5-10 and Luke 7:2-10)

Miracle number twelve appears in two gospels.

Matthew 8:5-10:

5. *Now when Jesus had entered Capernaum, a centurion came to Him, pleading with Him,*

6. *saying, "Lord, my servant is lying at home paralyzed, dreadfully tormented."*

7. *And Jesus said to him, "I will come and heal him."*

8. *The centurion answered and said, "Lord, I am not worthy that You should come under my roof. But only speak a word, and my servant will be healed.*

9. *"For I also am a man under authority, having soldiers under me. And I say to this one, 'Go,' and he goes; and to another, 'Come,' and he comes; and to my servant, 'Do this,' and he does it."*

10. *When Jesus heard it, He marveled, and said to those who followed, "Assuredly, I say to you, I have not found such great faith, not even in Israel!"*

Luke 7:2-10:

2. *And a certain centurion's servant, who was dear to him, was sick and ready to die.*

3. *So when he heard about Jesus, he sent elders of the Jews to Him, pleading with Him to come and heal his servant.*

4. *And when they came to Jesus, they begged Him earnestly, saying that the one for whom He should do this was worthy,*

5. *"for he loves our nation, and has built us a synagogue."*

6. *Then Jesus went with them. And when He was already not far from the house, the centurion sent friends to Him, saying to Him, "Lord, do not trouble Yourself, for I am not worthy that You should enter under my roof.*

7. *"Therefore I did not even think myself worthy to come to You. But say the word, and my servant will be healed.*

8. *"For I also am a man placed under authority, having soldiers under me. And I say to one, 'Go,' and he goes; and to another, 'Come,' and he comes; and to my servant, 'Do this,' and he does it."*

9. *When Jesus heard these things, He marveled at him, and turned around and said to the crowd that followed Him, "I say to you, I have not found such great faith, not even in Israel!"*

10. *And those who were sent, returning to the house, found the servant well who had been sick.*

This is a very famous story about the centurion and his servant who had come to Jesus telling Him that his servant was sick and Jesus said in Matthew 8:7: *"I will come and heal him. Verse 8: The centurion answered and said, "Lord, I am not worthy that You should come under my roof. But only speak a word, and my servant will be healed."*

This man had such a tremendous amount of faith, I'm sure Jesus saw the faith he had because He just simply said, "Go your way, and as you have believed it's going to happen."

If we could just get ourselves to the point where we really believe that Jesus does want us well, that Jesus does want us healed, that Jesus does want our employees healed, that Jesus does want our children healed and that Jesus does want our families healed, I think we would discover that we would all walk in a lot better health.

In the book of Luke it said that the servant was ready to die, but when his master heard of Jesus he immediately had faith and so he sent people to bring Jesus to him. (Apparently until that time he had not heard of Jesus.)

The same thing is true today. We have discovered as we go into foreign lands many people have never heard of Jesus, they have never heard of the healing power of God, they've never heard that God loves them and wants to make them well, and yet the minute they hear of it they come and are instantly healed.

I love Jesus' response when He said, *"I have not found such great faith, not even in Israel."* And yet, you'll notice that was the faith of a new person who had just heard about Jesus.

We oftentimes discover that people who are first born-again are the easiest ones to heal because their faith hasn't had an opportunity to get tainted, which it does so many times after we have been walking with Jesus for a while. We let doubt and unbelief come in instead of letting our faith grow stronger.

If your faith is "sagging", let someone who has real faith go after your healing for you!

MIRACLE NO. 13:
(Luke 7:11-15)

11. *Now it happened, the day after, that He went into a city called Nain; and many of His disciples went with Him, and a large crowd.*
12. *And when He came near the gate of the city, behold, a dead man was being carried out, the only son of his mother; and she was a widow. And a large crowd from the city was with her.*
13. *When the Lord saw her, He had compassion on her and said to her, "Do not weep."*
14. *Then He came and touched the open coffin, and those who carried him stood still. And He said, "Young man, I say to you, arise."*
15. *And he who was dead sat up and began to speak. And He presented him to his mother.*

This is the first time that the dead was raised in the ministry of Jesus, and yet there are only five short verses connected to this.

Isn't it amazing that such a tremendous miracle as raising the dead rates only five small verses in the Bible, and in only one book?

Probably the thing that stands out the most to me in this story is that Jesus had such compassion on the woman! It was because of this tremendous compassion for her losing what was apparently her only son that He spoke to the young man and said, "Arise."

You will notice that He did not speak to the mother, He spoke to the young man and the young man sat up, and there he was alive and well again!

As we race toward the end of time I believe we're going to see many more miracles of this type where the dead are raised. We just received a call the other day from some people in Burma who say that raising the dead is very common and very commonplace.

Benson Idahosa, a great man of Nigeria, had a most unusual conversion in that when he was saved, he instantly believed what the Bible said, that he could go out and lay hands on the sick and see them recover. He also believed that he could raise the dead! When you hear him tell this story it's absolutely fascinating because it shows a man who had incredible faith in salvation. He went up and down the streets looking for dead people; he'd knock at every door and say, "Is there any dead person in here? If there wasn't he would go on to the next.

He found eight dead people — the first one remained dead, the second one remained dead. The third one he said was deader than he was when he got there, but he didn't give up! I think this is so vital when we want to receive or maintain a healing or even raise the dead; we have to be persistent and we must not let go. He kept on going until he got to the eighth house — that person was raised from the dead!

Just imagine, a brand new convert who had just gotten saved and here he is out raising the dead. I believe that's one of the reasons today that Benson Idahosa is the man of God that he is, because he started out being persistent. You be persistent, too!

MIRACLE NO. 14:
(Matthew 12:22-23; Luke 11:14)

Matthew 12:22-23:

22. *Then one was brought to Him who was demon-possessed, blind and mute; and He healed him, so that the blind and mute man both spoke and saw.*

23. *And all the multitudes were amazed and said, "Could this be the Son of David?"*

Luke 11:14:

14. *And He was casting out a demon, and it was mute. So it was, when the demon had gone out, that the mute spoke; and the multitudes marveled.*

I want you to know that there is something very special about this particular miracle. A blind demoniac was cured and yet it rates two verses in Matthew and only one verse in Luke.

The man was blind, the man was dumb, and he both spoke and saw and yet that's all it rates in the Bible.

To me, this is an indication that healing is something we should expect to happen. You'll notice that the Bible doesn't write fifty pages on one little tiny healing, it just merely states a fact that they brought Him one that was possessed with a devil and He just cast the devils out, the devil of blindness, and the devil of dumbness.

It doesn't say a thing about the faith of the person involved, it merely said that when Jesus spoke the word, the devils came out and that same thing is true today! If we believe that Jesus is living on the inside of us we can use His name and devils will come out.

He is speaking to you today if you need a healing!

MIRACLE NO. 15:
(Matthew 8:23-27; Mark 4:35-40; Luke 8:22-25)

Matthew 8:23-27:

23. *Now when He got into a boat, His disciples followed Him.*
24. *And suddenly a great tempest arose on the sea, so that the boat was covered with the waves. But He was asleep.*
25. *Then His disciples came to Him and awoke Him, saying, "Lord, save us! We are perishing!"*
26. *But He said to them, "Why are you fearful, O you of little faith?" Then He arose and rebuked the winds and the sea. And there was a great calm.*
27. *And the men marveled, saying, "Who can this be, that even the winds and the sea obey Him?"*

Mark 4:35-40:

35. *On the same day, when evening had come, He said to them, "Let us cross over to the other side."*
36. *Now when they had left the multitude, they took Him along in the boat as He was. And other little boats were also with Him.*
37. *And a great windstorm arose, and the waves beat into the boat, so that it was already filling.*
38. *But He was in the stern, asleep on a pillow. And they awoke Him and said to Him, "Teacher, do You not care that we are perishing?"*
39. *Then He arose and rebuked the wind, and said to the sea, "Peace, be still!" And the wind*

ceased and there was a great calm.

40. *But He said to them, "Why are you so fearful? How is it that you have no faith?"*

Luke 8:22-25:

22. *Now it happened, on a certain day, that He got into a boat with His disciples. And He said to them, "Let us go over to the other side of the lake." And they launched out.*

23. *But as they sailed He fell asleep. And a windstorm came down on the lake, and they were filling with water, and were in jeopardy.*

24. *And they came to Him and awoke Him, saying, "Master, Master, we are perishing!" Then He arose and rebuked the wind and the raging of the water. And they ceased, and there was a calm.*

25. *But He said to them, "Where is your faith?" And they were afraid, and marveled, saying to one another, "Who can this be? For He commands even the winds and water, and they obey Him!"*

Panic, panic, panic! That's exactly what this miracle reminds me of! The disciples were trusting Jesus and were following Him along as He entered the ship. They were trustworthy and believing in Him for everything and believing that nothing was impossible with Him, and then what happened? Pow! A little bitty storm came up. Whether it was little or big, it can be exactly the same thing in our own personal lives, whether it's a financial crisis, whether it's a physical crisis, whether it's a marital crisis — regardless of what it is, suddenly our faith can go right out of our feet and we can become fearful, exactly like the disciples did at that time.

I wonder what went through the mind of Jesus at that time when He thought, "Here are these men who are supposed to really believe in Me and now suddenly just because a little storm comes up in their life they show they have not really learned to trust Me." Notice what He said to them, *"Where is your faith?"*

The biggest sin in the world today is still doubt and unbelief and it was that doubt and unbelief which came up in their lives! However, the thing I think is so tremendous is that while doubt and unbelief can keep us from receiving the miracles of God, in this particular instance He still went ahead and completed the miracle and calmed the sea.

It doesn't make any difference what the storm is in your life, it doesn't make any difference what you're going through right now — remember, Jesus is the One who can calm any storm.

Put your faith and trust in Him, and don't let doubt and unbelief sneak in, regardless of the circumstances!

MIRACLE NO. 16:
(Matthew 8:28-32; Mark 5:1-13; Luke 8:26-33)

Matthew 8:28-32:

28. *When He had come to the other side, to the country of the Gergesenes, there met Him two demon-possessed men, coming out of the tombs, exceedingly fierce, so that no one could pass that way.*

29. *And suddenly they cried out, saying, "What have we to do with You, Jesus, You Son of God? Have You come here to torment us before the time?"*

30. *Now a good way off from them there was a herd of many swine feeding.*

31. *So the demons begged Him, saying, "If You cast us out, permit us to go away into the herd of swine."*

32. *And He said to them, "Go." So when they had come out, they went into the herd of swine. And suddenly the whole herd of swine ran violently down the steep place into the sea, and perished in the water.*

Mark 5:1-13:

1. *Then they came to the other side of the sea, to the country of the Gadarenes.*

2. *And when He had come out of the boat, immediately there met Him out of the tombs a man with an unclean spirit,*

3. *who had his dwelling among the tombs; and no one could bind him, not even with chains,*

4. *because he had often been bound with shackles and chains. And the chains had been pulled apart by him, and the shackles broken in pieces; neither could anyone tame him.*

5. *And always, night and day, he was in the mountians and in the tombs, crying out and cutting himself with stones.*

6. *But when he saw Jesus from afar, he ran and worshiped Him.*

7. *And he cried out with a loud voice and said, "What have I to do with You, Jesus, Son of the Most High God? I implore You by God that You do not torment me."*

8. *For He said to him, "Come out of the man, unclean spirit!"*

9. *Then He asked him, "What is your name?" And he answered, saying, "My name is Legion; for we are many."*

10. *And he begged Him earnestly that He would not send them out of the country.*

11. *Now a large herd of swine was feeding there near the mountains.*

12. *And all the demons begged Him, saying, "Send us to the swine, that we may enter them."*

13. *And at once Jesus gave them permission. Then the unclean spirits went out and entered the swine (there were about two thousand); and the herd ran violently down the steep place into the sea, and drowned in the sea.*

Luke 8:26-33:

26. *Then they sailed to the country of the*

Gadarenes, which is opposite Galilee.

27. *And when He stepped out on the land, there met Him a certain man from the city who had demons for a long time. And he wore no clothes, nor did he live in a house but in the tombs.*

28. *When he saw Jesus, he cried out, fell down before Him, and with a loud voice said, "What have I to do with You, Jesus, Son of the Most High God? I beg You, do not torment me!"*

29. *For He had commanded the unclean spirit to come out of the man. For it had often seized him, and he was kept under guard, bound with chains and shackles; and he broke the bonds and was driven by the demon into the wilderness.*

30. *Jesus asked him, saying, "What is your name?" And he said, "Legion," because many demons had entered him.*

31. *And they begged Him that He would not command them to go out into the abyss.*

32. *Now a herd of many swine was feeding there on the mountain. And they begged Him that He would permit them to enter them. And He permitted them.*

33. *Then the demons went out of the man and entered the swine, and the herd ran violently down the steep place into the lake and drowned.*

This is another very interesting miracle, but aren't all of the miracles of Jesus interesting? You notice that He didn't specialize in just one type. He was capable of doing any and all kinds, and He is still capable today if we can remember, "He is the same yesterday, today and forever."

This is the famous story about the demoniac of Gadarenes. He was often bound with chains and fetters and he would just break them to pieces and no man could tame him. All day and all night he was in the mountains and he was in the tombs crying and cutting himself with stones.

But note that when Jesus was far off, this man ran and he did the same thing as the leper did in the book of Matthew the eighth chapter. He fell down first and worshiped Him.

If we could just remember to get our hearts in a position of worship which says, "Jesus, I love you with all of my heart and I believe that you will do the supernatural that I need done," I think we'd find ourselves receiving a lot more miracles.

This is the story where Jesus sent all of the demons into the swine and then they ran violently down a real steep mountain side and into the sea and drowned.

Each of the gospels tells a little different part about the man. You'll notice in the book of Luke it said that he wore no clothes nor did he live in any house but he lived in the tombs. You put all three of the stories together and you have a real good picture of a totally insane man. And yet, somehow or another the Spirit of God had penetrated his mind to make him believe that Jesus could do something for him. Isn't it unusual that the disciples were not afraid of the demon-possessed man until he was clothed and in his right mind; then the Bible tells us that they were afraid. We often wonder why people are afraid of the supernatural.

Could this be a reason that some people don't get healed because they really are afraid of the supernatural? I do not know the answer to that, I'm just asking you a question.

Some believe that this could possibly be two miracles even though the treatment and the situation was exactly the same. In Matthew the town was recorded as Gergesenes, and mentioned "two" men. Most theologians agree, however, that this was the same miracle, but differently recorded.

MIRACLE NO. 17:
(Matthew 9:20-22; Mark 5:25-34; Luke 8:43-48)

Matthew, Mark and Luke record miracle number seventeen which I think is one of the favorite stories of almost everybody, where the woman with the issue of blood was totally healed. This again was because of her tremendous faith.

Matthew 9:20-22:

20. *And suddenly, a woman who had a flow of blood for twelve years came from behind and touched the hem of His garment;*
21. *for she said to herself, "If only I may touch His garment, I shall be made well."*
22. *But Jesus turned around, and when He saw her He said, "Be of good cheer, daughter; your faith has made you well." And the woman was made well from that hour.*

Mark 5:25-34:

25. *Now a certain woman had a flow of blood for twelve years,*
26. *and had suffered many things from many physicians. She had spent all that she had and was no better, but rather grew worse.*
27. *When she heard about Jesus, she came behind Him in the crowd and touched His garment;*
28. *for she said, "If only I may touch His clothes, I shall be made well."*
29. *Immediately the fountain of her blood was dried up, and she felt in her body that she was healed of the affliction.*

30. *And Jesus, immediately knowing in Himself that power had gone out of Him, turned around in the crowd and said, "Who touched My clothes?"*

31. *But His disciples said to Him, "You see the multitude thronging You, and You say, 'Who touched Me?'"*

32. *And He looked around to see her who had done this thing.*

33. *But the woman, fearing and trembling, knowing what had happened to her, came and fell down before Him and told Him the whole truth.*

34. *And He said to her, "Daughter, your faith has made you well. Go in peace, and be healed of your affliction."*

Luke 8:43-48:

43. *Now a woman, having a flow of blood for twelve years, who had spent all her livelihood on physicians and could not be healed by any,*

44. *came from behind and touched the border of His garment. And immediately her flow of blood stopped.*

45. *And Jesus said, "Who touched Me?" When all denied it, Peter and those with him said, "Master, the multitudes throng You and press You, and You say, 'Who touched Me?'"*

46. *But Jesus said, "Somebody touched Me, for I perceived power going out from Me."*

47. *Now when the woman saw that she was not hidden, she came trembling; and falling down before Him, she declared to Him in the presence of*

all the people the reason she had touched Him and how she was healed immediately.

48. *And He said to her, "Daughter, be of good cheer; your faith has made you well. Go in peace."*

She had heard about the man Jesus, and I often think about what she went through to get to that man she had heard so much about.

She could have said, "I don't have any money to go because I spent it all on doctors."

She could also have said, "I am exhausted from having been sick so many years, there's no way I can possibly get to Him because He's so far away."

She also was unclean because she had an issue of blood and she could have really gotten into trouble going in public as a result of this.

There was such a tremendous crowd, she could have used that as an excuse for not getting to Jesus. But, nothing stopped her, absolutely nothing stopped her because all she kept saying was, "If I can just touch the hem of His garment, I'll be made whole."

Her faith was through touching something, but I believe her faith would have made her well regardless of whether she touched Him or not. I believe it was because of all the problems that she went through and the trouble that she went to to get to that one person whom she knew could heal her was what made her totally, instantly and completely healed. It's also very interesting to note that she did five things.

Number one — she heard.
Number two — she said.

Number three — she acted.

Number four — she received.

Number five — she told it.

If I were to pick out the two parts which I thought were the most important, it would be Number three and Number five.

She acted!

This is so vital because so many of us do not act.

Over and over again we have had people come up and ask us to pray for their mother or their father or their uncle or someone else and I'd say, "Well, are they here?" And they'll say, "No, they're too sick to come."

If you are too sick to come, that's when you need to be there!

You see, that's what she did — she acted, which is what so many people don't do, and Number five — she told it!

Every healing that God has ever given me, I have told it and have probably included it in some book or another along the line.

I believe that's one of the most important things in maintaining a healing is to keep telling people.

Luke 8:39: *"Return to your own house, and tell what great things God has done for you."*

This does not mean you're going to tell them when you *think* you're healed when you're not really healed, hoping that you can con God into doing it, but the minute you receive a legitimate healing, tell the world about it! That's what that woman did and that's why I believe that she received.

Another excellent point in that story is something that we all need to really look at in relation to our own life. Jesus said, "Somebody touched me." There were hundreds of people around Him and I'm sure that hundreds of people had brushed up against Him and had touched Him, but He said some very important words in Luke 8:46: *"Somebody touched me, for I perceived power going out from me."* That was an extremely interesting statement for Him to make because with all the other people touching Him, He did not feel the power going out of Him.

That's so easy to understand when you're in the healing ministry because we have been in what we call "hard audiences" which is where people have a lot of doubt and unbelief and skepticism and a determination to disprove the fact that God heals today. It's very difficult for miracles to happen under circumstances like that. However, we have also had many, many services, as a matter of fact, the bulk of our services are this way, where people come really expecting a miracle and they literally draw the power of God out of us and they get healed as a result.

Jesus did not feel the power go out of Him to anybody else until this woman touched Him and that was what made her whole. As the power went out of Him, He knew in His spirit that this woman had enough faith to make her whole and that's why it was so easy for the power to go out of Him into her!

MIRACLE NO. 18:
(Matthew 9:18, 23-25; Mark 5:22-23, 35-43; Luke 8:40-41, 49-56)

Matthew 9:18, 23-25:

18. *While He spoke these things to them, behold, a ruler came and worshiped Him, saying, "My daughter has just died, but come and lay Your hand on her and she will live."*

23. *And when Jesus came into the ruler's house, and saw the flute players and the noisy crowd wailing,*

24. *He said to them, "Make room, for the girl is not dead, but sleeping." And they laughed Him to scorn.*

25. *But when the crowd was put outside, He went in and took her by the hand, and the girl arose.*

Mark 5:22-23, 35-43:

22. *And behold, one of the rulers of the synagogue came, Jairus by name. And when he saw Him, he fell at His feet*

23. *and begged Him earnestly, saying, "My little daughter lies at the point of death. Come and lay Your hands on her, that she may be healed, and she will live."*

35. *While He was still speaking, some came from the ruler of the synagogue's house who said, "Your daughter is dead. Why trouble the Teacher any further?"*

36. *As soon as Jesus heard the word that was spoken, He said to the ruler of the synagogue, "Do*

not be afraid; only believe."

37. *And He permitted no one to follow Him except Peter, James, and John the brother of James.*

38. *Then He came to the house of the ruler of the synagogue, and saw a tumult and those who wept and wailed loudly.*

39. *When He came in, He said to them, "Why make this commotion and weep? The child is not dead, but sleeping."*

40. *And they laughed Him to scorn. But when He had put them all out, He took the father and the mother of the child, and those who were with Him, and entered where the child was lying.*

41. *Then He took the child by the hand, and said to her, "Talitha, cumi," which is translated, "Little girl, I say to you, arise."*

42. *Immediately the girl arose and walked, for she was twelve years of age. And they were overcome with great amazement.*

43. *But He commanded them strictly that no one should know it, and said that something should be given her to eat.*

Luke 8:40-41, 49-56:

40. *So it was, when Jesus returned, that the multitude welcomed Him, for they were all waiting for Him.*

41. *And behold, there came a man named Jairus, and he was a ruler of the synagogue. And he fell down at Jesus' feet and begged Him to come to his house.*

49. *While He was still speaking, someone came*

from the ruler of the synagogue's house, saying to him, "Your daughter is dead. Do not trouble the Teacher."

50. *But when Jesus heard it, He answered him, saying, "Do not be afraid; only believe, and she will be made well."*

51. *When He came into the house, He permitted no one to go in except Peter, James, and John, and the father and mother of the girl.*

52. *Now all wept and mourned for her; but He said, "Do not weep; she is not dead, but sleeping."*

53. *And they laughed Him to scorn, knowing that she was dead.*

54. *But He put them all out, took her by the hand and called, saying, "Little girl, arise."*

55. *Then her spirit returned, and she arose immediately. And He commanded that she be given something to eat.*

56. *And her parents were astonished, but He charged them to tell no one what had happened.*

The reason that this is so interesting is because one miracle is interrupted by another one happening. If you will recall, miracle number seventeen was the miracle of the woman with the issue of blood and the raising of Jairus' daughter was interrupted by the woman with the issue of blood.

There have been many times in our services when we will be laying hands on the sick and the Spirit of God will speak to us and tell us to go lay hands on someone else which in other words delays one person's miracle but is the exact instant God wants to do the first miracle.

This is a very interesting story because of that, and you will notice in all three of the gospels one miracle interrupts the story and then the circle comes back and picks up the story again.

One of the things that really breaks my heart in this story was in Matthew 9:24 where you'll notice that every one of the gospels say that they laughed when He said that she was not dead, but she was asleep.

The same thing is unfortunately true today where people will scorn any remark concerning the healing power of God.

We have seen this happen on television programs where the secular world does not understand and they laugh when you say, "In Jesus' name" or "Receive your healing in the name of Jesus."

Times haven't changed a single solitary bit. Jesus Christ is the same yesterday, today and forever and so the world laughed then, they still laugh today, but we win! Hallelujah!

Another very interesting point in these particular scriptures is that He "put them all out." When they laughed at Him, He put them all out.

Wouldn't it be wonderful if we had the courage and the boldness today to put out anybody who laughs when you begin to talk about the power of God. Just give us time and we'll do it.

Remember if there is an interruption or set back in your miracle, don't give up!

It's on the way!

MIRACLE NO. 19:
(Matthew 9:27-29)

The nineteenth miracle as remarkable as it is, appears in one gospel only.

27. *When Jesus departed from there, two blind men followed Him, crying out and saying, "Son of David, have mercy on us!"*

28. *And when He had come into the house, the blind men came to Him. And Jesus said to them, "Do you believe that I am able to do this?" They said to Him, "Yes, Lord."*

29. *Then He touched their eyes, saying, "According to your faith let it be to you."*

Three little verses and only three little verses are devoted to two blind men being healed. Let's look at what happens today when a blind person gets healed! I don't know about you, but Charles and I rejoice and rejoice and continue rejoicing.

We recently saw a young lady in Honduras who had been blinded at the age of four in one eye and when she was healed she didn't shut up for more than an hour. She was rejoicing and so exceedingly glad and yet, if you'll notice here are two blind men, obviously blind in both eyes, and Jesus just touched their eyes and He told them, "according to their faith," they could have their healing, and they were healed!

Isn't it wonderful when miracles can become so common that we can just say, "Well, praise the Lord. According to your faith be it unto you," and two blind people get healed.

MIRACLE NO. 20:
(Matthew 9:32-35)

A dumb demoniac healed is narrated in one gospel only!

32. *As they went out, behold, they brought to Him a man, mute and demon-possessed.*

33. *And when the demon was cast out, the mute spoke. And the multitudes marveled, saying, "It was never seen like this in Israel!"*

34. *But the Pharisees said, "He casts out demons by the ruler of the demons."*

35. *And Jesus went about all the cities and villages, teaching in their synagogues, preaching the gospel of the kingdom, and healing every sickness and every disease among the people.*

There are several unique points in these two verses of scripture. It merely says they brought the man to Him, and He cast the devil out. It doesn't say that he fought with the devil for hours and hours, and it didn't say that he "prayed" him out, but he cast the devil out. Then he promptly was accused of being of the devil. *The same thing happens today!* Don't worry, keep on casting out devils!

Devils need to be cast out! We need not fear a demonic spirit because Jesus gave us far more power than the devil. He said in Luke 10:19, *"Behold, I give you the authority to trample on serpents and scorpions, and over all the power of the enemy, and nothing shall by any means hurt you."*

He meant exactly what He said. That unlimited power He had was transferred to us and so we can cast out devils today as long as we believe that he meant what He said! We can even cast a spirit of infirmity out of ourselves if we have such a sickness. Simply speak the word to your own body!

MIRACLE NO. 21:
(Matthew 14:15-21; Mark 6:35-44;
Luke 9:12-17; John 6:5-13)

Miracle No. 21 concerns feeding the five thousand, and this particular miracle is extraordinary because it is narrated in all four gospels. Why this particular miracle registered strongly enough in the minds of Matthew, Mark, Luke and John is not known or even understood, except for the fact that it shows God's provision to multiply in an unlimited measure.

Matthew 14:15-21:

15. *When it was evening, His disciples came to Him, saying, "This is a deserted place, and the hour is already late. Send the multitudes away, that they may go into the villages and buy themselves food."*

16. *But Jesus said to them, "They do not need to go away. You give them something to eat."* (Notice that they were given permission to do this great miracle!)

17. *And they said to Him, "We have here only five loaves and two fish."*

18. *He said, "Bring them here to Me."*

19. *Then He commanded the multitudes to sit down on the grass. And He took the five loaves and the two fish, and looking up to heaven, He blessed and broke and gave the loaves to the disciples; and the disciples gave to the multitudes.*

20. *So they all ate and were filled, and they took up*

twelve baskets full of the fragments that re-mained.

21. *Now those who had eaten were about five thousand men, besides women and children.*

Mark 6:35-44:

35. *And when the day was now far spent, His disciples came to Him and said, "This is a deserted place, and already the hour is late.*

36. *"Send them away, that they may go into the surrounding country and villages and buy themselves bread; for they have nothing to eat."*

37. *But He answered and said to them, "You give them something to eat." And they said to Him, "Shall we go and buy two hundred denarii worth of bread and give them something to eat?"*

38. *But He said to them, "How many loaves do you have? Go and see." And when they found out they said, "Five, and two fish."*

39. *Then He commanded them to make them all sit down in groups on the green grass.*

40. *So they sat down in ranks, in hundreds and in fifties.*

41. *And when He had taken the five loaves and the two fish, He looked up to heaven, blessed and broke the loaves, and gave them to His disciples to set before them; and the two fish He divided among them all.*

42. *So they all ate and were filled.*

43. *And they took up twelve baskets full of fragments and of the fish.*

44. *Now those who had eaten the loaves were about five thousand men.*

Luke 9:12-17:

12. *When the day began to wear away, the twelve came and said to Him, "Send the multitude away, that they may go into the surrounding towns and country, and lodge and get provisions; for we are in a deserted place here."*
13. *But He said to them, "You give them something to eat." And they said, "We have no more than five loaves and two fish, unless we go and buy food for all these people."*
14. *For there were about five thousand men. And He said to His disciples, "Make them sit down in groups of fifty."*
15. *And they did so, and made them all sit down.*
16. *Then He took the five loaves and the two fish, and looking up to heaven, He blessed and broke them, and gave them to the disciples to set before the multitude.*
17. *So they all ate and were filled, and twelve baskets of the leftover fragments were taken up by them.*

John 6:5-13:

5. *Then Jesus lifted up His eyes, and seeing a great multitude coming toward Him, He said to Philip, "Where shall we buy bread, that these may eat?"*
6. *But this He said to test him, for He Himself knew what He would do.*
7. *Philip answered Him, "Two hundred denarii*

worth of bread is not sufficient for them, that every one of them may have a little."

8. *One of His disciples, Andrew, Simon Peter's brother, said to Him,*

9. *"There is a lad here who has five barley loaves and two small fish, but what are they among so many?"*

10. *Then Jesus said, "Make the people sit down." Now there was much grass in the place. So the men sat down, in number about five thousand.*

11. *And Jesus took the loaves, and when He had given thanks He distributed them to the disciples, and the disciples to those sitting down; and likewise of the fish, as much as they wanted.*

12. *So when they were filled, He said to His disciples, "Gather up the fragments that remain, so that nothing is lost."*

13. *Therefore they gathered them up, and filled twelve baskets with the fragments of the five barley loaves which were left over by those who had eaten.*

Read all four of these examples with the idea in mind that even if you should be one of five thousand sick, God always has provision for you. He knows about you, even though there may be millions who are also sick, and He can make the special provision you need for your illness.

And the wonderful thing is — there is always enough healing power left over to heal everyone else. If you will note, there was more left over than they started with!

That's God compassion!

MIRACLE NO. 22:
(Matthew 14:22-32; Mark 6:48-50; John 6:16-21)

Matthew 14:22-32:

22. *Immediately Jesus made His disciples get into the boat and go before Him to the other side, while He sent the multitudes away.*
23. *And when He had sent the multitudes away, he went up on a mountain by Himself to pray. And when evening had come, He was alone there.*
24. *But the boat was now in the middle of the sea, tossed by the waves, for the wind was contrary.*
25. *Now in the fourth watch of the night Jesus went to them, walking on the sea.*
26. *And when the disciples saw Him walking on the sea, they were troubled, saying, "It is a ghost!" And they cried out for fear.*
27. *But immediately Jesus spoke to them, saying, "Be of good cheer! It is I; do not be afraid."*
28. *And Peter answered Him and said, "Lord, if it is You, command me to come to You on the water."*
29. *So He said, "Come." And when Peter had come down out of the boat, he walked on the water to go to Jesus.*
30. *But when he saw that the wind was boisterous, he was afraid; and beginning to sink he cried out, saying, "Lord, save me!"*
31. *And immediately Jesus stretched out His hand and caught him, and said to him, "O you of litle faith, why did you doubt?"*
32. *And when they got into the boat, the wind ceased.*

Mark 6:48-50:

48. *Then he saw them straining at rowing, for the wind was against them. And about the fourth watch of the night He came to them, walking on the sea, and would have passed them by.*

49. *But when they saw Him walking on the sea, they supposed it was a ghost, and cried out;*

50. *for they all saw Him and were troubled. And immediately He talked with them and said to them, "Be of good cheer! It is I; do not be afraid."*

John 6:16-21:

16. *And when evening came, His disciples went down to the sea,*

17. *got into the boat, and went over the sea toward Capernaum. And it was now dark, and Jesus had not come to them.*

18. *Then the sea arose because a great wind was blowing.*

19. *So when they had rowed about three or four miles, they saw Jesus walking on the sea and drawing near the boat; and they were afraid.*

20. *But He said to them, "It is I; do not be afraid."*

21. *Then they willingly received Him into the boat, and immediately the boat was at the land where they were going.*

This story is full of miracles and other points for us to remember in dealing with sickness, although this story does not concern sickness at all.

First, Jesus walked on the water.

Second, Peter walked on the water.

Third, Peter began to sink.

Fourth, Jesus brought him into the boat, and immediately they were on the land!

Applying this to your healing, there are times when we need to walk on spiritual water. We need to let our faith stretch out further than ever before.

This is what Peter did, and in your case, if it is a healing for which you're believing, or have received and are still questioning, when Peter put his eyes on the circumstances, he lost what he had gained with faith. When the miracle was done, they were immediately on shore.

Consider this — you start to get worse, Jesus reaches down and touches you, and immediately you are healed!

MIRACLE NO. 23:
(Matthew 15:21-28; Mark 7:25-29)

Miracle No. 23 concerns the healing of the Syro-Phoenician woman's daughter, and is narrated in two gospels.

Matthew 15:21-28:

21. *Then Jesus went out from there and departed to the region of Tyre and Sidon.*

22. *And behold, a woman of Canaan came from that region and cried out to Him, saying, "Have mercy on me, O Lord, Son of David! My daughter is severely demon-possessed."*

23. *But He answered her not a word. And His disciples came and urged Him, saying, "Send her away, for she cries out after us."*

24. *But He answered and said, "I was not sent except to the lost sheep of the house of Israel."*

25. *Then she came and worshiped Him, saying, "Lord, help me!"*

26. *But He answered and said, "It is not good to take the children's bread and throw it to the little dogs."*

27. *And she said, "True, Lord, yet even the little dogs eat the crumbs which fall from their masters' table."*

28. *Then Jesus answered and said to her, "O woman, great is your faith! Let it be to you as you desire." And her daughter was healed from that very hour.*

Mark 7:25-29:

25. *For a woman whose young daughter had an unclean spirit heard about Him, and she came and fell at His feet.*
26. *The woman was a Greek, a Syro-Phoenician by birth, and she kept asking Him to cast the demon out of her daughter.*
27. *But Jesus said to her, "Let the children be filled first, for it is not good to take the children's bread and throw it to the little dogs."*
28. *And she answered and said to Him, "Yes, Lord, yet even the little dogs under the table eat from the children's crumbs."*
29. *Then He said to her, "For this saying go your way; the demon has gone out of your daughter."*

This story particularly fascinates me because of the woman's persistence, which I personally believe is one of the greatest helps in receiving a healing and also in maintaining it.

The second thing she did was to worship Him, saying, "Lord, help me!" She admitted that she needed something far more than she could do in the natural. Even though Jesus did not immediately answer her, when He saw her persistence which He saw as a faith that would not stop, He granted her the desire of her heart. We need to keep our faith out there with persistence until we receive what we need!

Don't give up!

MIRACLE NO. 24:
(Mark 7:32-37)

Miracle No. 24 shows the healing of the deaf and dumb man.

32. *Then they brought to Him one who was deaf and had an impediment in his speech, and they begged Him to put His hand on him.*

33. *And He took him aside from the multitude, and put His fingers in his ears, and He spat and touched his tongue.*

34. *Then, looking up to heaven, He sighed, and said to him, "Ephphatha," that is, "Be opened."*

35. *Immediately his ears were opened, and the impediment of his tongue was loosed, and he spoke plainly.*

36. *Then He commanded them that they should tell no one; but the more He commanded them, the more widely they proclaimed it.*

37. *And they were astonished beyond measure, saying, "He has done all things well. He makes both the deaf to hear and the mute to speak.*

One of the things that surprises me about this scripture is that it is recorded in only one gospel. Notice in this miracle that the man did not come by himself, but he was brought by friends. Norma Jean LeRoy, about whom we wrote the book IMPOSSI-BLE MIRACLES, was brought by friends, although as she says, she was "dragged!" The faith of friends when you might not have any, can be a tremendous help in receiving a healing!

Notice that Jesus healed in many different ways!

MIRACLE NO. 25:
(Matthew 15:32-38; Mark 8:1-9)

Miracle No. 25 concerns the feeding of the four thousand, and is contained in two gospels.

Matthew 15:32-38:

32. *Then Jesus called His disciples to Him and said, "I have compassion on the multitude, because they have now continued with Me three days and have nothing to eat. And I do not want to send them away hungry, lest they faint on the way."*

33. *Then His disciples said to Him, "Where could we get enough bread in the wilderness to fill such a great multitude?"*

34. *Jesus said to them, "How many loaves do you have?" And they said, "Seven, and a few little fish."*

35. *And He commanded the multitude to sit down on the ground.*

36. *And He took the seven loaves and the fish and gave thanks, broke them and gave them to His disciples; and the disciples gave to the multitude.*

37. *So they all ate and were filled, and they took up seven large baskets full of the fragments that were left.*

38. *Now those who ate were four thousand men, besides women and children.*

Mark 8:1-9:

1. *In those days, the multitude being very great and having nothing to eat, Jesus called His disciples to Him and said to them,*
2. *"I have compassion on the multitude, because they have now been with Me three days and have nothing to eat.*
3. *"And if I send them away hungry to their own houses, they will faint on the way; for some of them have come from afar."*
4. *Then His disciples answered Him, "How can one satisy these people with bread here in the wilderness?"*
5. *He asked them, "How many loaves do you have?" And they said, "Seven."*
6. *And He commanded the multitude to sit down on the ground. And He took the seven loaves and gave thanks, broke them and gave them to His disciples to set before them; and they set them before the multitude.*
7. *And they had a few small fish; and having blessed them, He said to set them also before them.*
8. *So they ate and were filled, and they took up seven large baskets of leftover fragments.*
9. *Now those who had eaten were about four thousand. And He sent them away.*

This miracle shows how Jesus overcame all the doubts of the disciples. Oftentimes in our families we will have those who will preach doom and gloom concerning our healing. Remember your own faith can help you out of a lot of situations, even though they may not look bright at the moment.

Notice also in this miracle that Jesus *gave away the provision and when He gave*, it was multiplied. It wasn't multiplied until He gave away what He had! Again, note that He had more when He finished than when He started!

When we "give away" healing by laying hands on the sick, it is amazing how our own healings will multiply!

MIRACLE NO. 26:
(Mark 8:22-25)

Miracle No. 26 concerns the blind man of Bethsaida being healed, and this miraculous healing is narrated in only one gospel.

22. *Then He came to Bethsaida; and they brought a blind man to Him, and begged Him to touch him.*
23. *So He took the blind man by the hand and led him out of the town. And when He had spit on his eyes and put His hands on him, He asked him if he saw anything.*
24. *And he looked up and said, "I see men like trees, walking."*
25. *Then He put His hands on his eyes again and made him look up. And he was restored and saw everyone clearly.*

Again this is a story of friends who brought a blind man to Jesus and they (not the blind man) asked for his healing! This is an unusual healing, but when I read it, I always think it is God showing His sovereignty by doing it exactly as He wants it done.

Jesus touched the man again when he said he could only see men as trees, showing that we need not be ashamed to go back more than once for our healing.

This does not show a lack of faith, but persistence!

MIRACLE NO. 27:
(Matthew 17:14-21; Mark 9:17-29; Luke 9:38-42)

Miracle No. 27 concerns the healing of an epileptic child, and is related in three gospels.

Matthew 17:14-21:

14. *And when they had come to the multitude, a man came to Him, kneeling down to Him and saying,*
15. *"Lord, have mercy on my son, for he is an epileptic and suffers severely; for he often falls into the fire and often into the water.*
16. *So I brought him to Your disciples, but they could not cure him."*
17. *Then Jesus answered and said, "O faithless and perverse generation, how long shall I be with you? How long shall I bear with you? Bring him here to Me."*
18. *And Jesus rebuked the demon, and he came out of him; and the child was cured from that very hour.*
19. *Then the disciples came to Jesus privately and said, "Why could we not cast him out?"*
20. *So Jesus said to them, "Because of your unbelief; for assuredly, I say to you, if you have faith as a mustard seed, you will say to this mountain, 'Move from here to there,' and it will move; and nothing will be impossible for you.*
21. *However, this kind does not go out except by prayer and fasting."*

Mark 9:17-29:

17. *Then one from the multitude answered and said, "Teacher, I brought You my son, who has a mute spirit.*

18. *And wherever he seizes him, he throws him down; he foams at the mouth, gnashes his teeth, and becomes rigid. So I spoke to Your disciples, that they should cast him out, but they could not."*

19. *He answered him and said, "O faithless generation, how long shall I be with you? How long shall I bear with you? Bring him to Me."*

20. *Then they brought him to Him. And when he saw Him, immediately the spirit convulsed him, and he fell on the ground and wallowed, foaming at the mouth.*

21. *So He asked his father, "How long has this been happening to him?" And he said, "From childhood.*

22. *"And often he has thrown him both into the fire and into the water to destroy him. But if You can do anything, have compassion on us and help us."*

23. *Jesus said to him, "If you can believe, all things are possible to him who believes."*

24. *Immediately the father of the child cried out and said with tears, "Lord, I believe; help my unbelief!"*

25. *When Jesus saw that the people came running together, He rebuked the unclean spirit, saying to him, "You deaf and dumb spirit, I command you, come out of him, and enter*

him no more!"

26. *Then the spirit cried out, convulsed him greatly, and came out of him. And he became as one dead, so that many said, "He is dead."*

27. *But Jesus took him by the hand and lifted him up, and he arose.*

28. *And when He had come into the house, His disciples asked Him privately, "Why could we not cast him out?"*

29. *So He said to them, "This kind can come out by nothing but prayer and fasting."*

Luke 9:38-42:

38. *Suddenly a man from the multitude cried out, saying, "Teacher, I implore You, look on my son, for he is my only child.*

39. *"And behold, a spirit seizes him, and suddenly cries out; it convulses him so that he foams at the mouth, and bruising him, it departs from him with great difficulty.*

40. *"So I implored Your disciples to cast it out, but they could not."*

41. *Then Jesus answered and said, "O faithless and perverse generation, how long shall I be with you and bear with you? Bring your son here."*

42. *And as he was still coming, the demon threw him down and convulsed him. Then Jesus rebuked the unclean spirit, healed the child, and gave him back to his father.*

The father of this child brought him and told Jesus that His disciples could not cast the spirit out, and Jesus rebuked them, and went on and set the child free. In this story is one of the most powerful of all the scriptures, *"If you can believe, all things are possible to him who believes"* (Mark 9:23).

But the heartbreaking thing is the father's reply, *"Lord, I believe; help my unbelief!"* (Mark 9:24). Many of us are in that same position right now — we believe (to a point) and we need to ask Jesus to help our unbelief. But also note that Jesus healed the boy in spite of the father's unbelief.

MIRACLE NO. 28:
(Matthew 17:24-27)

Miracle No. 28 concerns finding money in the mouth of a fish, and as remarkable as this story is, it is found only in this one gospel. No other gospel relates the story.

24. *And when they had come to Capernaum, those who received the temple tax came to Peter and said, "Does your Teacher not pay the temple tax?"*

25. *He said, "Yes." And when he had come into the house, Jesus anticipated him, saying, "What do you think, Simon? From whom do the kings of the earth take customs or taxes, from their own sons or from strangers?"*

26. *Peter said to Him, "From strangers." Jesus said to him, "Then the sons are free.*

27. *Nevertheless, lest we offend them, go to the sea, cast in a hook, and take the fish that comes up first. And when you have opened its mouth, you will find a piece of money; take that and give it to them for Me and you."*

How many fish swim around with money in their mouth? Not many, and yet the very first fish that Peter caught was the one Jesus was talking about! He had cold, hard cash in his mouth, enough to pay the taxes.

Jesus can accomplish the healing of your problem from many different sources, so just be obedient to Him and expect a miracle!

MIRACLE NO. 29:
(John 9:1-41)

Miracle No. 29, narrated in only one gospel is the story of the man born blind.

1. *Now as Jesus passed by, He saw a man who was blind from birth.*
2. *And His disciples asked Him, saying, "Rabbi, who sinned, this man or his parents, that he was born blind?"*
3. *Jesus answered, "Neither this man nor his parents sinned, but that the works of God should be revealed in him.*
4. *"I must work the works of Him who sent Me while it is day; the night is coming when no one can work.*
5. *"As long as I am in the world, I am the light of the world."*
6. *When He had said these things, He spat on the ground and made clay with the saliva; and He anointed the eyes of the blind man with the clay.*
7. *And He said to him, "Go, wash in the pool of Siloam" (which is translated, Sent). So he went and washed, and came back seeing.*
8. *Therefore the neighbors and those who previously had seen that he was blind said, "Is not this he who sat and begged?"*
9. *Some said, "This is he." Others said, "He is like him." He said, "I am he."*
10. *Therefore they said to him, "How were your eyes opened?"*

11. *He answered and said, "A Man called Jesus made clay and anointed my eyes and said to me, 'Go to the pool of Siloam and wash.' So I went and washed, and I received sight."*
12. *Then they said to him, "Where is He?" He said, "I do not know."*
13. *They brought him who formerly was blind to the Pharisees.*
14. *Now it was a Sabbath when Jesus made the clay and opened his eyes.*
15. *Then the Pharisees also asked him again how he had received his sight. He said to them, He put clay on my eyes, and I washed, and I see."*
16. *Therefore some of the Pharisees said, "This Man is not from God, because He does not keep the Sabbath." Others said, "How can a man who is a sinner do such signs?" And there was a division among them.*
17. *They said to the blind man again, "What do you say about Him because He opened your eyes?" He said, "He is a prophet."*
18. *But the Jews did not believe concerning him, that he had been blind and received his sight, until they called the parents of him who had received his sight.*
19. *And they asked them, saying, "Is this your son, who you say was born blind? How then does he now see?"*
20. *His parents answered them and said, "We know that this is our son, and that he was born blind;*
21. *"but by what means he now sees we do not know, or who opened his eyes we do not know.*

He is of age; ask him. He will speak for himself."

22. *His parents said these things because they feared the Jews, for the Jews had agreed already that if anyone confesssed that He was Christ, he would be put out of the synagogue.*

23. *Therefore his parents said, "He is of age; ask him."*

24. *So they again called the man who was blind, and said to him, "Give God the glory! We know that this Man is a sinner."*

25. *He answered and said, "Whether He is a sinner or not I do not know. One thing I know: that though I was blind, now I see."*

26. *Then they said to him again, "What did He do to you? How did He open your eyes?"*

27. *He answered them, "I told you already, and you did not listen. Why do you want to hear it again? Do you also want to become His disciples?"*

28. *Then they reviled him and said, "You are His disciple, but we are Moses' disciples.*

29. *"We know that God spoke to Moses; as for this fellow, we do not know where He is from."*

30. *The man answered and said to them, "Why, this is a marvelous thing, that you do not know where He is from, and yet He has opened my eyes!*

31. *"Now we know that God does not hear sinners; but if anyone is a worshiper of God and does His will, He hears him.*

32. *"Since the world began it has been unheard of that anyone opened the eyes of one who was born blind.*

33. *"If this Man were not from God, He could no nothing."*
34. *They answered and said to him, "You were completely born in sins, and are you teaching us?" And they cast him out.*
35. *Jesus heard that they had cast him out; and when He had found him, He said to him, "Do you believe in the Son of God?"*
36. *He answered and said, "Who is He, Lord, that I may believe in Him?"*
37. *And Jesus said to him, "You have both seen Him and it is He who is talking with you."*
38. *Then he said, "Lord, I believe!" And he worshiped Him.*
39. *And Jesus said, "For judgment I have come into this world, that those who do not see may see, and that those who see may be made blind."*
40. *Then some of the Pharisees who were with Him heard these words, and said to Him, "Are we blind also?"*
41. *Jesus said to them, "If you were blind, you would have no sin; but now you say, 'We see.' Therefore your sin remains.*

This remarkable story brings up an interesting question, "Is sickness due to the sin of parents or the individual himself?" Jesus' answer eliminated the question.

The second most important part was he obeyed Jesus when he told him to go and wash in the pool of Siloam. He did just what Jesus said, and he came back seeing.

But there were skeptics there, just as there are

today! They questioned how it was done, and even called the parents of the child who had received his sight. Then the Pharisees called Jesus a sinner because He did miracles on Sunday.

A thing to remember in your own healing when people question if it is the devil, is what the blind man answered in verse 25: *He answered and said, "Whether He is a sinner or not I do not know. One thing I know: that though I was blind, now I see."*

MIRACLE NO. 30:
(Luke 13:11-17)

Miracle No. 30 is another of the great miracles of the Bible which is told in only one gospel, and yet what a wonderful miracle it is!

11. *And behold, there was a woman who had a spirit of infirmity eighteen years, and was bent over and could in no way raise herself up.*

12. *But when Jesus saw her, He called her to Him and said to her, "Woman, you are loosed from your infirmity."*

13. *And He laid His hands on her, and immediately she was made straight, and glorified God.*

14. *But the ruler of the synagogue answered with indignation, because Jesus had healed on the Sabbath; and he said to the crowd, "There are six days on which men ought to work; therefore come and be healed on them, and not on the Sabbath day."*

15. *The Lord then answered him and said, "Hypocrite! Does not each one of you on the Sabbath loose his ox or his donkey from the stall, and lead it away to water it?*

16. *"So ought not this woman, being a daughter of Abraham, whom Satan has bound—think of it— for eighteen years, be loosed from this bond on the Sabbath?"*

17. *And when He said these things, all His adversaries were put to shame; and all the multitude rejoiced for all the glorious things that were done by Him.*

This woman, who apparently had arthritis or osteoporosis had been bent over for eighteen years. When Jesus spoke to her, she was instantly made whole and she glorified God, BUT the rulers of the synagogue again said Jesus was of the devil because he healed on the Sabbath day, however when He answered in verse 16, even his adversaries were ashamed!

This story always reminds me of one of the first big miracles which happened in one of our earlier meetings.

Shortly after we received the baptism with the Holy Spirit, we went on a visit to a church who did not know we had received! I was going to give a short little talk on how to make the Bible come alive, but as were were driving to the location, God spoke and said, "I want you to share that healing is for today!"

What a day of miracles it was, but the one we remember the most is the lady with osteoporosis who was bent over so far that you could not see anything but her back as she came down the aisle! We spoke healing to her, and she fell under the power of God with a tremendous "crack", but when she stood up she was inches taller! No longer was there a "hump" on her back, she was as straight as an arrow!

She was about 70 years old, and had been sitting on the front pew of her church for years because she was so bent over she could not get in the pews, and on Sunday morning she was still in the same place sitting straight up! Her pastor did not believe in healing and his sermon that morning was entitled "Healing is not for today!"

Every time he said that statement, she said, "Hallelujah!"

He continued, "Healing is of the devil," and she answered, "Hallelujah!"

We went back to the same place years later and she was still perfectly healed! Hallelujah!

Have you noticed in almost every miracle that the devil is right there to try to steal, kill and destroy? Whenever the devil comes at you and tells you your healing is not from God, stomp on him quickly and remind him whom you serve!

. . .And remember, we have more power than the devil.

MIRACLE NO. 31:
(Luke 14:1-6)

Miracle No. 31 is narrated in only one gospel. It concerns the man who had dropsy which is also known as edema, or an excessive amount of fluid in the body which causes extreme swelling.

1. *Now it happened, as He went into the house of one of the rulers of the Pharisees to eat bread on the Sabbath, that they watched Him closely.*
2. *And behold, there was a certain man before Him who had dropsy.*
3. *And Jesus, answering, spoke to the lawyers and Pharisees, saying, "Is it lawful to heal on the Sabbath?"*
4. *But they kept silent. And He took him and healed him, and let him go.*
5. *Then He answered them, saying, "Which of you, having a donkey or an ox that has fallen into a pit, will not immediately pull him out on the Sabbath day?"*
6. *And they could not answer Him regarding these things.*

Jesus got to the question before the Pharisees asked him, and He asked them in verse 3, *"Is it lawful to heal on the Sabbath?"* They didn't answer him, and Jesus took the man and healed him, and let him go. Then He asked them the question about retrieving an animal which had fallen in a pit on the Sabbath, but they couldn't give Him a good answer.

This miracle doesn't tell how the fluid left the man's body, but is another example of how nothing is impossible with God! But it was a miracle which they could see, because it was an instant healing.

Again, notice that the devil was right there with his "theology". Pay no attention to him!

I remember one time in California, there was a sovereign move of God and one man came forward and as we asked him what his miracle was, he said, "I just lost thirty-five pounds!" He had been singing in the choir, and as the power of God enveloped the auditorium, he sovereignly lost about 35 pounds of fluid, or weight, and his huge stomach was now flat!

Ignore the devil and watch God work in your life.

MIRACLE NO. 32:
(Luke 17:11-19)

Miracle No. 32 is again narrated in one gospel only. This is where Jesus healed the ten lepers.

11. *Now it happened as He went to Jerusalem that He passed through the midst of Samaria and Galilee.*

12. *Then as He entered a certain village, there met Him ten men who were lepers, who stood afar off.*

13. *And they lifted up their voices and said, "Jesus, Master, have mercy on us!"*

14. *So when He saw them, He said to them, "Go, show yourselves to the priests." And so it was that as they went, they were cleansed.*

15. *Now one of them, when he saw that he was healed, returned, and with a loud voice glorified God,*

16. *and fell down on his face at His feet, giving Him thanks. And he was a Samaritan.*

17. *So Jesus answered and said, "Were there not ten cleansed? But where are the nine?*

18. *Were there not any found who returned to give glory to God except this foreigner?"*

19. *And He said to him, "Arise, go your way. Your faith has made you well."*

Jesus is recorded as healing 10 lepers. Their opening statement is "Jesus, Master, have mercy on us". (Cry of desperation) Then Jesus instructs them to "test their faith" by going and "showing yourselves to the priests". Now, as they turned to go, they were not yet healed. And if they arrived at the priests' house with the signs of leprosy they would not only look foolish, but would be in trouble. But the word says that "as they were going, they were cleansed".

Now, look at the power of the "heart of thanksgiving." One of them turned to really express his gratitude to Jesus. The word says that he "fell on his face at His feet, giving thanks to Him! As a result of this extra heart-felt thanksgiving, he was "made whole" which means that even all the eaten off parts were restored.

I thank Him every day for what He has done in my life simply because I am grateful to be alive and well, but I also believe that is a great part in maintaining what God has given you!

MIRACLE NO. 33:
(John 11:1-44)

Miracle No. 33, the raising of Lazarus from the dead is told in one gospel only. John thought this was worthy of recording, or maybe he was the only one there!

1. *"Now a certain man was sick, Lazarus of Bethany, the town of Mary and her sister Martha.*

2. *It was that Mary who anointed the Lord with fragrant oil and wiped His feet with her hair, whose brother Lazarus was sick.*

3. *Therefore the sisters sent to Him, saying, "Lord, behold, he whom You love is sick."*

4. *When Jesus heard that, He said, "This sickness is not unto death, but for the glory of God, that the Son of God may be glorified through it."*

5. *Now Jesus loved Martha and her sister and Lazarus.*

6. *So, when He heard that he was sick, He stayed two more days in the place where He was.*

7. *Then after this He said to the disciples, "Let us go to Judea again."*

8. *The disciples said to Him, "Rabbi, lately the Jews sought to stone You, and are You going there again?"*

9. *Jesus answered, "Are there not twelve hours in the day? If anyone walks in the day, he does not stumble, because he sees the light of this world.*

10. *"But if one walks in the night, he stumbles, because the light is not in him."*

11. *These things He said, and after that He said to them, "Our friend Lazarus sleeps, but I go that I may wake him up."*

12. *Then His disciples said, "Lord, if he sleeps he will get well."*

13. *However, Jesus spoke of his death, but they thought that He was speaking about taking rest in sleep.*

14. *Then Jesus said to them plainly, "Lazarus is dead.*

15. *"And I am glad for your sakes that I was not there, that you may believe. Nevertheless let us go to him."*

16. *Then Thomas, who is called Didymus, said to his fellow disciples, "Let us also go, that we may die with Him."*

17. *So when Jesus came, He found that he had already been in the tomb four days.*

18. *Now Bethany was near Jerusalem, about two miles away.*

19. *And many of the Jews had joined the women around Martha and Mary, to comfort them concerning their brother.*

20. *Then Martha, as soon as she heard that Jesus was coming, went and met Him, but Mary was sitting in the house.*

21. *Then Martha said to Jesus, "Lord, if You had been here, my brother would not have died.*

22. *"But even now I know that whatever You ask of God, God will give You."*

23. *Jesus said to her, "Your brother will rise again."*

24. *Martha said to Him, "I know that he will rise again in the resurrection at the last day."*
25. *Jesus said to her, "I am the resurrection and the life. He who believes in Me, though he may die, he shall live.*
26. *"And whoever lives and believes in Me shall never die. Do you believe this?"*
27. *She said to Him, "Yes, Lord, I believe that You are the Christ, the Son of God, who is to come into the world."*
28. *And when she had said these things, she went her way and secretly called Mary her sister, saying, "The Teacher has come and is calling for you."*
29. *As soon as she heard that, she arose quickly and came to Him.*
30. *Now Jesus had not yet come into the town, but was in the place where Martha met Him.*
31. *Then the Jews who were with her in the house, and comforting her, when they saw that Mary rose up quickly and went out, followed her, saying, "She is going to the tomb to weep there."*
32. *Then, when Mary came where Jesus was, and saw Him, she fell down at His feet, saying to Him, "Lord, if You had been here, my brother would not have died."*
33. *Therefore, when Jesus saw her weeping, and the Jews who came with her weeping, He groaned in the spirit and was troubled.*
34. *And He said, "Where have you laid him?" They said to Him, "Lord, come and see."*
35. *Jesus wept.*

36. *Then the Jews said, "See how He loved him!"*
37. *And some of them said, "Could not this Man, who opened the eyes of the blind, also have kept this man from dying?"*
38. *Then Jesus, again groaning in Himself, came to the tomb. It was a cave, and a stone lay against it.*
39. *Jesus said, "Take away the stone." Martha, the sister of him who was dead, said to Him, "Lord, by this time there is a stench, for he has been dead four days."*
40. *Jesus said to her, "Did I not say to you that if you would believe you would see the glory of God?"*
41. *Then they took away the stone from the place where the dead man was lying. And Jesus lifted up His eyes and said, "Father, I thank You that You have heard Me.*
42. *"And I know that You always hear Me, but because of the people who are standing by I said this, that they may believe that You sent Me."*
43. *Now when He had said these things, He cried with a loud voice, "Lazarus, come forth!"*
44. *And he who had died came out bound hand and foot with graveclothes, and his face was wrapped with a cloth. Jesus said to them, "Loose him, and let him go."*

Jesus actually put off the raising of Lazarus for forty-eight hours because when the word reached Him that Lazarus was dead, He stayed two days longer where He was. Sometimes we get impatient and want our healing "right now" but this shows me that Jesus does it in His perfect timing.

It always amazes me the way Jesus ministered healing so easily and without fanfare.

One of the most significant things about this story is that Martha had faith in the fact Lazarus would not have died if Jesus had been there, and she knew he would be raised in the resurrection, but it is amazing that she didn't have the faith for a NOW miracle! The same fact remains today. People believe that Jesus CAN do it but they're not sure He WILL do it now.

Believe for your miracle NOW!

MIRACLE NO. 34:
(Matthew 20:30-34; Mark 10:46-52; Luke 18:35-43)

Miracle No. 34 concerns healing blind Bartimaeus, and while this is told in three gospels, only Matthew records there were two blind men healed!

Matthew 20:30-34:

30. *And behold, two blind men sitting by the road, when they heard that Jesus was passing by, cried out, saying, "Have mercy on us, O Lord, Son of David!"*

31. *Then the multitude warned them that they should be quiet; but they cried out all the more, saying, "Have mercy on us, O Lord, son of David!"*

32. *So Jesus stood still and called them, and said, "What do you want Me to do for you?"*

33. *They said to Him, "Lord, that our eyes may be opened."*

34. *So Jesus had compassion and touched their eyes. And immediately their eyes received sight, and they followed Him.*

Mark 10:46-52:

46. *Then they came to Jericho. And as He went out of Jericho with His disciples and a great multitude, blind Bartimaeus, the son of Timaeus, sat by the road begging.*

47. *And when he heard that it was Jesus of Nazareth, he began to cry out and say, "Jesus, Son of David, have mercy on me!"*

48. *Then many warned him to be quiet; but he cried out all the more, "Son of David, have mercy on me!"*

49. *So Jesus stood still and commanded him to be called. Then they called the blind man, saying to him, "Be of good cheer. Rise, He is calling you."*

50. *And throwing aside his garment, he rose and came to Jesus.*

51. *And Jesus answered and said to him, "What do you want Me to do for you?"*

52. *The blind man said to Him, "Rabboni, that I may receive my sight." Then Jesus said to him, "Go your way; your faith has made you well." And immediately he received his sight and followed Jesus on the road.*

When Bartimaeus heard that Jesus was coming his way he cried out, *"Jesus, Son of David, have mercy on me!"* When he was told that Jesus was calling him the word says that *"throwing aside his garment, he rose up, and came to Jesus"*.

This is an act of faith for a blind man. Jesus spoke the word of healing, he was healed, and *"followed him, glorifying God: and all the people, when they saw it, gave praise unto God"* (Luke 18:43 KJV).

Luke 18:35-43:

35. *Then it happened, that as He was coming near Jericho, that a certain blind man sat by the road begging.*

36. *And hearing a multitude passing by, he asked what it meant.*

37. *So they told him that Jesus of Nazareth was passing by.*
38. *And he cried out, saying, "Jesus, Son of David, have mercy on me!"*
39. *Then those who went before warned him that he should be quiet; but he cried out all the more, "Son of David, have mercy on me!"*
40. *So Jesus stood still and commanded him to be brought to Him. And when he had come near, He asked him,*
41. *saying, "What do you want Me to do for you?" And he said, "Lord, that I may receive my sight."*
42. *Then Jesus said to him, "Receive your sight; your faith has saved you."*
43. *And immediately he received his sight, and followed Him, glorifying God. And all the people, when they saw it, gave praise to God.*

Humanity of writers — told it as they saw and heard and they told it from memory. Accurate but not religious in exactness. They didn't get together and compare their writing, but all were confirming one another. Notice the different ways three writers told the story: Luke said that he was coming near Jericho and Jesus wanted the blind man brought to him. Matthew said they were departing from Jericho and Jesus called them to Him. Mark said as they went out of Jericho, Jesus commanded him to be called.

There is something in each of these thirty-seven miracles that is just for you. The part that I like is that the blind man immediately followed

Jesus, glorifying God. Also, ALL the people, when they saw it, gave praise to God.

We can never give God too much praise.

MIRACLE NO. 35:
(Matthew 21:18-22; Mark 11:12-14; 20-26)

Miracle No. 35 concerns the cursing of the fig tree which is related in two gospels.

Matthew 21:18-22:

18. *Now in the morning, as He returned to the city, He was hungry.*

19. *And seeing a fig tree by the road, He came to it and found nothing on it but leaves, and said to it, "Let no fruit grow on you ever again." And immediately the fig tree withered away.*

20. *Now when the disciples saw it, they marveled, saying, "How did the fig tree wither away so soon?"*

21. *So Jesus answered and said to them, "Assuredly, I say to you, if you have faith and do not doubt, you will not only do what was done to the fig tree, but also if you say to this mountain, 'Be removed and be cast into the sea,' it will be done.*

22. *And all things, whatever you ask in prayer, believing, you will receive."*

Mark 11:12-14; 20-26:

12. *Now the next day, when they had come out from Bethany, He was hungry.*

13. *And seeing from afar a fig tree having leaves, He went to see if perhaps He would find something on it. And when he came to it, He found nothing but leaves, for it was not the season for figs.*

14. *In response Jesus said to it, "Let no one eat fruit from you ever again." And His disciples heard*

it.
20. *Now in the morning, as they passed by, they saw the fig tree dried up from the roots.*
21. *And Peter, remembering, said to Him, "Rabbi, look! The fig tree which You cursed has withered away."*
22. *So Jesus answered and said to them, "Have faith in God.*
23. *"For assuredly, I say to you, whoever says to this mountain, 'Be removed and be cast into the sea,' and does not doubt in his heart, but believes that those things he says will come to pass, he will have whatever he says.*
24. *"Therefore I say to you, whatever things you ask when you pray, believe that you receive them, and you will have them.*
25. *"And whenever you stand praying, if you have anything against anyone, forgive him, that your Father in heaven may also forgive you your trespasses.*
26. *"But if you do not forgive, neither will your Father in heaven forgive your trespasses."*

Notice here also, how differently each writer described and worded the lesson, but the message was made clear.

Almost every miracle that Jesus did makes me realize or reminds me of the fact that absolutely nothing is impossible with God if we can just believe, not that it CAN happen, but that it WILL happen. This is one of the most important things to remember in receiving a healing.

Probably the reason this is a favorite of mine is

a similar miracle that happened to us many years ago and was included in a little book called THERE IS POWER IN THE NAME OF JESUS!

"...*and his name shall be called Wonderful, Counsellor, The Mighty God, The Everlasting Father, The Prince of Peace*" (Isa. 9:6 KJV). That is what we should call Him at all times. His NAME IS Wonderful, Counsellor, The mighty God, The Everlasting Father, The Prince of Peace!" His NAME IS ALL in all and over all, except God himself!

"*Worthy is the Lamb that was slain to receive power, and riches, and wisdom, and strength, and honour, and glory, and blessing*" (Rev. 5:12 KJV).

This is how we should look at the name of Jesus, as the name is full of power and riches, and wisdom, and strength, and honour, and glory, and blessing!

I think of the innumerable times we have called on the NAME of Jesus! Sometimes for BIG things, and many times for small things, but He has always been faithful to the Word which says His name is above every other name.

We were in Connecticut one year during tobacco growing time. I had never seen tobacco grown in the field, and didn't know that it could look absolutely beautiful and lush and green. As we came into the city and noticed all these beautiful fields, many of which were growing under what looked like a huge gauze covering, I inquired of the cab driver what they were.

He told me it was tobacco!

When the Lord delivered me of cigarettes right

after I was saved, I understood the problems of people who depend on cigarettes for a number of things, including nerves, weight, fear, etc., and at that time he gave me a ministry to loose people from this bondage of the devil.

All I could see in those beautiful fields of green were hundreds, thousands and probably even millions of cigarettes.

I remembered the story of Jesus and the fig tree and how the fig tree withered! I prayed a quick prayer and said, "Father, in the NAME of Jesus, I ask you to wither those tobacco plants, wither them, wither them, wither them!"

The next morning I came out of the Tobacco Valley Inn (what a name for the motel they put us in) and the tobacco plants were flourishing, so once again I prayed, "In Jesus' NAME, wither them, wither them, wither them, Father."

The next morning the plants were still flourishing, so I prayed the same prayer again, "In the NAME of Jesus, Father, wither those tobacco plants, wither those tobacco plants!"

When we left town three days later, the plants were still thriving, but about two weeks after we got home, we received several letters which said, "Did you hear about the tornado which swept through this area, uprooting all the tobacco plants, and now they are lying out in the sun, withering away!"

Hallelujah! There's POWER in the NAME of Jesus! (Special note: We immediately asked God to replace the tobacco crops with an even more profitable crop so the farmers wouldn't lose out!)

Even though this miracle is only in two of the gospels, it has some of the greatest scriptures and revelation. Mark 11:23 and 24 can put a charge into your life. A lot of detail on this is shared in the book HOW TO HEAL THE SICK.

Mark 11:25 goes into one of the greatest hindrances to healing — and that is unforgiveness. A lot more detail on this subject is told in the special chapter in this book on forgiveness.

This story reminds me of a woman who came to one of our services with a baby in her womb which seventeen gynecologists had told her to abort! The baby had no kidneys, no stomach, and two lungs which would never develop!

She came to one of our services believing that if we laid hands on her, her baby would be made normal!

What a mountain she faced, and yet she came and did not doubt in her heart one single bit, but believed that the things which she had said would come to pass!

How right she was! Six months later we held her beautiful little boy in our arms at a Healing Explosion and he has two perfect kidneys, two lungs that operate normally, and a perfect stomach.

Remember whatever your problem is, God is bigger than your problem!

Get your expectors up!

MIRACLE NO. 36:
(Luke 22:50-52)

Miracle No. 36 concerns a creative miracle and that is the restoration of Malchus' ear when Peter cut it off.

50. *And one of them struck the servant of the high priest and cut off his right ear.*

51. *But Jesus answered and said, "Permit even this." And He touched his ear and healed him.*

52. *Then Jesus said to the chief priests, captains of the temple, and the elders who had come to Him, "Have you come out, as against a robber, with swords and clubs?"*

Proof again that nothing is impossible with God, even to the restoration of something that has been cut off. He has the best "Elmer's glue" of anyone I know.

MIRACLE NO. 37:
(John 21:1-14)

Miracle No. 37 is narrated in this one gospel and is an after-resurrection miracle.

1. *After these things Jesus showed Himself again to the disciples at the Sea of Tiberias, and in this way He showed Himself:*
2. *Simon Peter, Thomas called Didymus, Nathanael of Cana in Galilee, the sons of Zebedee, and two others of His disciples were together.*
3. *Simon Peter said to them, "I am going fishing." They said to him, "We are going with you also." They went out and immediately got into the boat, and that night they caught nothing.*
4. *But when the morning had now come, Jesus stood on the shore; yet the disciples did not know that it was Jesus.*
5. *Then Jesus said to them, "Children, have you any food?" They answered Him, "No."*
6. *And He said to them, "Cast the net on the right side of the boat, and you will find some." So they cast, and now they were not able to draw it in because of the multitude of fish.*
7. *Therefore that disciple whom Jesus loved said to Peter, "It is the Lord!" Now when Simon Peter heard that it was the Lord, he put on his outer garment (for he had removed it), and plunged into the sea.*

8. *But the other disciples came in the little boat (for they were not far from land, but about two hundred cubits), dragging the net with fish.*

9. *Then, as soon as they had come to land, they saw a fire of coals there, and fish laid on it, and bread.*

10. *Jesus said to them, "Bring some of the fish which you have just caught."*

11. *Simon Peter went up and dragged the net to land, full of large fish, one hundred and fifty-three; and although there were so many, the net was not broken.*

12. *Jesus said to them, "Come and eat breakfast." Yet none of the disciples dared ask Him, "Who are You?—knowing that it was the Lord.*

13. *Jesus than came and took the bread and gave it to them, and likewise the fish.*

14. *This is now the third time Jesus showed Himself to His disciples after He was raised from the dead.*

This concerns changing the position of your faith. They had fished all night, caught nothing, and Jesus told them to put their net down on the other side of the boat.

Sometimes we keep fishing in the same place for our healing. Maybe we have had the same people praying for us. Let's get out and get into another spirit-filled meeting. Maybe someone there will know something new and different about healing your type of illness, or have a special gift of faith (better results) in a particular kind of healing.

Sometimes Charles gets people healed for

whom I have prayed; other times I succeed after he has ministered with no results.

I have a real specialty for barren women. My faith is 100% in this area. I was looking at a picture of a physician this morning who had a sterile sperm and came to one of our meetings and in ten months he had a beautiful little boy. They now have two. My faith was at top level when I laid hands on him and commanded a supernatural sperm to form in him.

Charles' real specialty is in backs. He is the one who calls the examples up on the stage, and we have seen the most impossible situations healed when he ministers. Both of us have tremendous faith in back problems, yet at times neither of us will have success and later on we will hear that someone who has taken our training will succeed!

You will notice when Simon Peter obeyed, the net was full and they had an immediate fish fry. You should immediately have an instant praise celebration when you receive your healing.

Jesus apparently never prayed at the temple gate for the lame man, but Peter and John later did. Perhaps the timing for God's purpose is divinely selected and not according to us!

Perhaps Jesus saved this man's healing to show Peter and John that they could do miracles, just like He's telling us today!

3   The Name of Jesus Rings Bells

As vital as anything else in receiving and maintaining a healing, is to believe in the power that resides in the name of Jesus! When we first hear about Jesus, it is strictly "head" knowledge, but when we receive a revelation from God it becomes "heart" knowledge.

We need to believe with the *heart* that the name of Jesus is above cancer, rheumatoid arthritis, diabetes, heart problems, multiple sclerosis, cerebral palsy and any other disease known and unknown to man. It cannot only be head knowledge, it has to get down into the heart.

The NAME of Jesus brought forth some of the greatest miracles in the Bible, and is still doing the same thing today. Peter and John were walking by the temple one day when they saw the lame man sitting there. *Then Peter said, "Silver and gold I do not have, but what I do have I give you: In the name of Jesus Christ of Nazareth, rise up and walk"* (Acts

3:6). And the man walked! Peter had no more natural power than you or I have, but he used the supernatural name that was available to him. He used the name of Jesus!

This is the first time Peter ever used the name of Jesus as a tool for healing. Jesus had told them that they could use His name to do whatever miracles needed to be done, but up until this point it was strictly "head" knowledge!

Jesus had said, "I give you the right to use my name!"

"I give you power of attorney to use my name!"

"Use it for whatever circumstances you need to use it. And as often as you like, and as many times as you like!

Peter looked at the crippled man, and what did he see? What did he perceive?

He perceived that the man had faith to be healed! Suddenly revelation knowledge began working in Peter. He looked into this man's eyes and saw something he had never seen before. He probably thought, "Wow, this guy's expecting to be healed. That's really neat, but how do I do it? What do I do now? I don't have faith for his healing. What am I going to do because this man's expecting a miracle!"

Then the revelation knowledge not only began working, it became a reality as Peter said, "Silver and gold I do not have, but such as I have..." and the revelation knowledge hit Peter like a ton of bricks! I imagine bells began ringing! — ding, ding, ding,

ding!

What do I have?

What do I have?

I have all the power that's in the name of Jesus! I have ALL power in heaven and earth because it was given to Him and He turned around and gave it to me! That wonderful revelation knowledge hit Peter, and it went from his head to his heart, that he actually did have all power in heaven and earth!

There was that special moment of revelation when he realized that Jesus meant it when He said, "I give YOU power to tread on serpents and scorpions." That's when he said (and believed it), "In the name of Jesus Christ of Nazareth, rise up and walk!" Glory to God — it worked! It worked!

You can walk up to a hundred wheelchairs and say, "Silver and gold have I none, but such as I have, I give unto thee, in the name of Jesus Christ of Nazareth, rise up and walk," but until you get that revelation knowledge, it will not be effective.

And what do you really have? You have the same resurrection power in you that brought the Lord Jesus Christ right out of the grave when you have the baptism with the Holy Spirit.

You've got the name that is above every other name.

You've got the name that is above every disease.

You've got the name which makes the devil tremble when you use it.

When I got that revelation years ago, my Bible suddenly said, "Frances Hunter, all power in heaven and earth is given unto me. Now, Frances Hunter, I give it to you."

I remembered a song we sang many years ago, "Oh, to be His hand extended, reaching out to the oppressed." He said, "You ARE my hand extended!" I looked at my hand with those funny little brown spots on it and thought, "How about that? That's the hand of Jesus!" And revelation knowledge went straight as an arrow into my heart!

The minute YOU get that revelation in your spirit, the minute that YOU believe that ALL power in heaven and earth belongs to YOU, you're on your way to a miracle!

We were in a city in Florida and a lady came up on the stage with a metastasized cancer on her cheek. She had a huge, hard lump on her face. I walked over to her and started to say, "In the name of Jesus," but before I got the words out, I touched it!

Jesus had said, "Those are not your hands, Frances Hunter, they are mine!" And before I even got out the words, "In the name of Jesus," that big metastasized cancer turned to jelly, and I began pushing on the thing because I wondered where it had gone? I expected it to go, but not that fast!

There was a doctor sitting on the stage with me and he screamed, "I saw it! I saw it!"

...But this is even more interesting!

I have a letter from him and he said, "I just wanted to double check on you, so I went and checked out that lady after the service, and there's not a sign of cancer left!"

We are not a powerless church, and we do not have a powerless gospel.

We are not powerless people. We are people who have the power of God!

"For I am not ashamed of the gospel of Christ, for it is the POWER of God!"

4   Stay In The Word!

I love to read the Bible!

It is loaded with promises direct from the heart of God.

It can change the course of your life, your happiness and your health if you will just absorb what it says!

There is healing in the Word of God, and the more you familiarize yourself with what it says, the better your position is to receive what you need and want from God. Psalm 46 is a scripture I use often in my own life, and it can be used in yours to receive or keep your healing. This is the way my Bible reads:

GOD (and that one word alone can accomplish miracles) *is Frances Hunter's refuge and strength.*

A very PRESENT (not past or future, but in the NOW) *help in trouble.*

(Therefore Frances Hunter will not fear),
Though the earth be removed,
(Frances Hunter will not fear)
And though the mountains be carried into the midst of the sea;

(Frances Hunter will not fear)
Though its waters roar and be troubled,
(Frances Hunter will not fear)
Though the mountains shake with its swelling.
(Frances Hunter will not fear!)

Put your own name in there, regardless of how sick you are, what the prognosis is for your life or your physical body, say it over and over and OVER, and see the results it produces! Whatever situation you are in right now physically, remember that God is a very PRESENT help in time of your trouble!

It's good to read more than one version of the Bible! We have a copy of practically every Bible that has been printed, and we refer to all of them.

Some of the best advice concerning maintaining a healing is contained in I Chronicles 16:8-11. Here are three different versions. The Living Bible says:

8. *"Oh, give thanks to the Lord and pray to him,"*
   they sang.
   "Tell the peoples of the world
   About his mighty doings.
9. *Sing to him; yes, sing his praises*
   And tell of his marvelous works.
10. *Glory in his holy name;*
    Let all rejoice who seek the Lord.
11. *Seek the Lord; yes, seek his strength*
    And seek his face UNTIRINGLY.

The New King James Version gives a little different wording:

8. *Oh, give thanks to the Lord!*
   Call upon His name;

Make known His deeds among the peoples!
9. *Sing to Him, sing psalms to Him;*
   Talk of all His wondrous works!
10. *Glory in His holy name;*
    Let the hearts of those rejoice who seek the LORD!
11. *Seek the LORD and His strength;*
    Seek His face EVERMORE!

And for those who like the King James Version, here's what it says:

8. *Give thanks unto the Lord, call upon his name, make known his deeds among the people.*
9. *Sing unto him, sing psalms unto him, talk ye of all his wondrous works.*
10. *Glory ye in his holy name: let the heart of them rejoice that seek the Lord.*
11. *Seek the Lord and his strength, seek his face CONTINUALLY.*

As you will note, in all three versions we are commanded to do several things:

1. Give thanks unto the Lord
2. Call upon His name
3. Make known His deeds among men
4. Sing unto Him
5. Sing psalms unto Him
6. Talk of all His wondrous works
7. Glory in His holy name
8. Let the hearts of seekers rejoice
9. Seek the Lord
10. Seek His strength
11. Seek His face CONTINUALLY, EVERMORE, UNTIRINGLY

There is no way I can ever impress upon you enough the necessity and privilege of thanking God for what He has done in your life. Call upon His name over and over in the event the devil tries to give you back what you were healed of!

Give a testimony as often as you can of His deeds, praise Him, and talk of everything He has done for you.

Glory in His name, and seek Him continually, evermore and UNTIRINGLY!

John 8:31,32 says: *"If you abide in My word, you are My disciples indeed. And you shall know the truth, and the truth shall make you free"* (NKJV).

"Then said Jesus to those Jews which believed on him, 'If ye CONTINUE in my word, then are ye my disciples indeed; And ye shall know the truth, and the truth shall make you free" (KJV).

The word "abide" means to dwell, reside, live, stay, submit to — so if we stay in His word, submit to it, literally reside in it, and let it live in us, then we shall know the truth and the truth shall make us free!

Continue simply means, "Don't stop!" So we need to stay in His word, because it doesn't say that just because you've read a portion of scripture, or even the entire Bible that you should stop. We need to grow daily in the Lord, not just an occasional day, but every single day of our lives! Through this we can become more healthy spiritually, emotionally and physically!

Psalm 34:1 says, *"I will bless the Lord at all times; His praise shall continually be in my mouth."*

Your praises are a sweet smelling fragrance unto the Lord, and He loves smelling that sweetness!

Bury the Word of God in your heart and keep it there for receiving and maintaining a healing!

When the situation looks bad, begin to laugh. "A merry heart doeth good like a medicine" (Proverbs 17:22 KJV), so meditate on the Word of God.

I love Jeremiah 32:27. *"Behold, I am the Lord, the God of all flesh. Is there anything too hard for Me?"* No! Is it too hard for God to heal a disease from which no one has ever been healed before? No. We say, "That's easy! "

Remember that it is when you meditate on the Word of God that you understand your position in God. When you understand, that's when you can stand!

Proverbs 4:4 says, *Let your heart RETAIN my words; Keep my commands, and LIVE.*

Proverbs 4:20-22 says,

20. *"My son, give attention to my words;*
    Incline your ear to my sayings.
21. *Do not let them depart from your eyes;*
    Keep them in the midst of your heart;
22. *For they are LIFE to those who find them,*
    And HEALTH to all their flesh!

    I shall not die, but live,
And declare the works of the Lord (Psalms 118:17).

O Lord my God, I cried out to You,
And You have healed me (Psalms 30:1,2).

Sometimes we have a feeling there is no way out, over or under where our problems are concerned, and here's a fabulous verse for any situation, including sickness. Again, quoting the handwritten things in my Bible, this is what it says:

Fear not, for I (God) *have redeemed you* (Frances Hunter);

I have called you by your name (Frances Hunter);

You, (Frances Hunter) *are Mine.*

When you pass through the waters,

I, God, will be with you, (Frances Hunter)

And through the rivers,

(Frances Hunter), *they shall not overflow you.*

(Frances Hunter), *when you walk through the fire,*

You shall not be burned.

Nor shall the flame scorch you, (Frances).

For I am the Lord your God, The Holy One of Israel, your Savior.

(Isaiah 43:1-3).

Put your name in where I have placed mine, and see what it does for you personally!

Remember, He'll be with you through fire and water, and you'll not drown, nor will you be burned. That's a promise of God!

I want to encourage you to go through the Bible searching for verses that speak to you personally about your own healing! It's wonderful what God will do to highlight scriptures perfect for your understanding and situation!

You might be thinking about this time, "Why do I need to know how to receive and maintain a healing? I'm not sick!" Let me assure you that you never know when the devil is going to come in and take a poke at you. You will notice today that the people who are being attacked the most are the ones in God's army who are on the front lines.

The devil doesn't have to worry about the pew-sitters. They're doing nothing. It's the ones who are out there on the front line that he really attacks. That is why it is vital, because the very fact that you are reading this book tells me that you have come off of the back lines and gone into the front line! Stay there, but stay healthy!

5 Maintaining Is As Important As Receiving

Receiving a healing is one of the most important things in the world, especially if you are the one who is sick.

It is interesting in ministering healing that we can do the same thing to one person that we do to you and it might not work on them and it might work on you.

What's the difference? One is ready to receive a healing, and the other is not.

What makes a person ready? First, you need to be in a receptive mood. You need to put your "expectors" up, anticipating to receive when hands are laid on you.

The most vital thing you have to know is that it *is* God's will for you to be well. God wants us to walk in divine health, so when we have to receive a healing, we are accepting second best, but second best is better than first worst! Isn't it wonderful to know that in the event we don't always walk in divine health, we can receive a healing for whatever our problem is?

The most important thing, I believe, is not necessarily big faith, but just enough faith to believe that God wants you well. As I shared with you previously, the thing that kept me from being concerned about how sick I was, was the fact that I KNEW God wanted me well.

I KNEW that God wasn't finished with me.

I KNEW that the ministry to which God had called me was not completed yet, so I was never concerned about dying.

I want to share with you something else that I believe had a lot to do with my receiving my healing.

I never complained!

I believe this is where many people get themselves in trouble, because the minute they get sick, they say, "Why me, God? Why me?"

You have no idea how disastrous it was to our ministry when I was off for six weeks. Charles had to go out on his own all alone, and we're not used to that! The two of us are used to always ministering together and are called by God to minister as one, but we knew that he had to go, even if I couldn't go with him.

I could have bellowed all over the place and said, "God, how come you had to do this to me?" "Why did you have to pick on me?" "You know how busy I am for the kingdom of God." "Why did you have to do this to me?"

That never entered my mind. God could have prevented what the devil laid on me, and why He did not, I do not know, nor do I care. All I know is that He healed me. But all the time I was lying in bed, I never complained to God. I didn't gripe about a single solitary thing. I just listened to some Holy Ghost tapes and waited until God's timing was for me.

Did you ever meet a Christian who complained about everything? "Well, I don't know why God had to allow this to happen or that to happen." I believe when you begin to talk like that, you are taking yourself out of a position where God will be able to heal you.

Did you also notice as you read the story of my "incurable" sickness, that I did not get healed INSTANTLY? I spent six miserable weeks flat on my back.

When Charles prayed for me the first time, I expected to get well! I could have said to Charles, "What's the matter with you?" It's very interesting that almost every other time Charles has laid hands on me, I have received an instant healing once he knew exactly what was wrong.

He laid hands on me for a new heart May 14, 1974, and God gave me a brand new heart instantly! My blood pressure was 225/140, and it went down in twelve minutes to 140/80 and it has stayed there ever since. I just had a heart echo made, and the heart echo is as perfect as anything you ever saw. When God does it, God does it! BUT...hang on to it.

Now, how do you hang on to a healing?

"The thief cometh not, but for to steal, to kill, and to destroy" (John 10:10 KJV). But Jesus says, "I

have come to give you life, and life more abundantly."

The minute you get healed, the devil will come in and will try to convince you that you didn't get healed. More people lose their healings through doubt and unbelief than any other way I know.

I have seen many people who get healed in a service go back to their seat, and their good Christian brother, good Christian sister, good Christian husband or wife throw a big arrow of doubt, and will say, "Are you sure you got healed?" "Try and see if you can't find some pain."

Who's talking? The devil! It's not your husband. It's not your wife. It's not your brother or sister. It's the devil who is talking to you, and he is trying to plant a thought in your mind that you didn't really get healed.

Do you know what happens? I've seen people do things that would give me a pain (and I'm healthy) if I tried to do some of the crazy things they do. It sometimes seems as if they are trying to encourage it to return. Also, remember this — you didn't get sick in a split second, so give God a little more time! We have seen many healings take place overnight, even though nothing was apparent at the time of laying on of hands.

The best way to receive a healing and to keep it is to say, "Thank you, Jesus. Thank you, Jesus. Thank you, Jesus. Thank you, Jesus." For some reason, those are the hardest three words in the world for people to say. I cannot understand that. But the minute you say, "Thank you, Jesus," what you are really also saying is, "I got it! I got it! I latched onto it!" That's why I always say, "Thank you, Jesus," without any consideration of whether I got healed or not. To me, it is an automatic response to say, "Thank you, Jesus." So many times, we don't thank Him, but continue to look for the sickness!

A good thing to remember is, "Don't look for the sickness, look for the healing. Don't look for the pain, look for the lack of pain, or even the reduction of pain.

I personally believe the greatest way to maintain a healing is to give a testimony of your healing. Every time God has healed me, I have shouted it from the housetop! I've had to write a book about it. Hallelujah!

Every time you give a testimony of your own healing, it is going to confirm it right back to you. After I was healed of endocarditis, I shared the very next night in San Antonio, and praise the Lord I have my words on video!

What happened next?

The devil came charging right after me!

How?

I did not realize that my immune system was basically totally destroyed during that illness. I did not realize how easy it would be for me to catch something else after that. We went to the Long Beach Healing Explosion in California. Everybody on our team, believe it or not, got a virus that was almost in epidemic stage in Long Beach.

You never saw a sadder looking group of people coming back from a Healing Explosion than all these great people on the healing teams. We were all sick as could be, and couldn't wait to get home. Of course, since all of my body systems were down, I got it worse than anyone else.

I went to bed as soon as I got home and stayed there for about 10 days. Now let me show you what your good Christian friends do unknowingly: "Frances, are you sure you got healed?" "Are you sure that it's not that same thing back on you?"

You have no idea how many telephone calls I received like that. Everyone of them said, "Are you sure it's not the same thing back on you?" And I said, "On November 8, 1988, God healed me and God doeth all things well. No, this is not the same thing back again. This is just the good old Long Beach virus that I brought home along with everybody else."

They weren't concerned about anyone else but they said, "Probably that same thing is back on you." And I said, "No, it is not."

Do you see what I did? I didn't listen to the garbage that was being put in my ears. I could have listened to it and I could have thought, "That probably is the truth. That infection has probably gotten back into my blood stream again. I'll probably die this time."

I said, "No, this is *not* the same thing." I added, "This is just a virus that I've caught and I'll get over this and I'll feel fine."

I recovered in time and felt wonderful and went to New Haven to the Healing Explosion. They had an unexpected change in the weather; it went below freezing and guess what I caught? A cold! I had not had a cold in more than ten years but this one was horrible! I was so hoarse on the day of the Healing Explosion, I could hardly talk!

We came home. Again, I went to bed, and again I got telephone calls! "See, I told you that you didn't get healed. Are you sure this isn't that same thing?"

I said, "No, I've just got a cold. I haven't had a cold in ten years but for some reason or another I've got a cold, but I'm catching a healing."

Suddenly Charles and I remembered when we were little kids growing up that our mother or daddy said to us, "Your resistance is low. Your resistance is run down and I don't want you to get your resistance down because that is when you get a cold."

Charles said, "Your resistance (immune system) is down because of your having been sick."

Then he said, "You need a new immune system!"

He immediately prayed for a new immune system for me. I am thoroughly convinced that the immune system plays one of the greatest roles in keeping our bodies healthy.

Today, when I lay hands on anyone, regardless of their problem, I speak a new immune system into them. When plagued with various or numerous illnessess, we need to remember our immune system needs to be boosted at all times. When your immune system is low or destroyed, you are open to every disease that comes along.

A few years ago everybody thought that when

you had an immune system deficiency, you had Aids. That is not true! People with rheumatoid arthritis have a low or no immune system. That is why they cannot throw off that horrible disease.

People with cancer need a new immune system.

Any physical body that has an "incurable" disease needs a new immune system.

"When a body is ill, it is not always fighting off foreign invaders. Some diseases occur when the immune system becomes confused and stops functioning, or actually attacks the body's own cells. Allergies strike when the immune system overreacts to ordinarily harmless substances like dust or the droplet of toxin in a bee sting, causing inflammation. Multiple sclerosis results from immune cells damaging the central nervous system, causing tingling, blindness and paralysis. Rheumatoid arthritis can be one of the more severe types of arthritis. Immune cells attack and inflame the joints and surrounding soft tissue, causing pain and deformity." (From the U.S. News & World Report, July 2, 1990).

Remember, "The thief comes not but for to steal, to kill and destroy." I do not know of anyone whom the devil has not visited after a healing.

Even though God gave me a new heart in 1974, every so often the devil tries to put a pain in my heart. I lay my hand on my heart and say, "Devil, get lost!" Then I remind him, "May 14th, 1974, God gave me a brand new heart."

The devil immediately takes off because He can't stand it when you throw the truth at him!

Give your testimony often of being healed. That will get you away from doubt and unbelief.

Two of the greatest things which will steal your healing are doubt and unbelief. All these well-meaning friends who speak doubt and unbelief into you can rob you of your healing.

Use common sense. I've seen people who were healed of diabetes who immediately went out and went on a dessert binge just to see if they really got healed. That's foolishness!

When I was healed of diabetes, I went three years without ever tasting sugar because I thought that was great wisdom. Now I eat sugar moderately and it doesn't phase me a single solitary bit. But please use common sense after a healing.

Use wisdom and get plenty of rest and sleep. Have you ever found yourself susceptible to a cold when you stayed up (even to do good things) until 2 o'clock in the morning at a prayer meeting? It was really wonderful and you were just having the greatest time, the Spirit of God was moving and then you got a cold as a result! God intends for you to use common sense, wisdom and normal health rules.

When we first started in the ministry, we had Bible studies in our house. All of our Healing Explosions started from a little Bible study in our house. When the clock struck 12, we said, "Out in the name of Jesus." And we meant it! We literally ran everybody out of the house.

I believe the devil goes to work at 12:01. I can't really say that because Charles and I were married at 12:01 in the morning on New Year's Day of 1970, so I'll say the devil goes to work at 12:02!

Stand on the Word of God. There has never failed one word of all the good promises of God.

Psalm 27:5 (KJV) says, *"For in the time of trouble he shall hide me in his pavilion; in the secret of his tabernacle shall he hide me; he shall set me up upon a rock."*

I will never be moved. You cannot shake my faith one minute concerning the fact that God healed me on November 8, 1988 of an incurable disease. I know that I know that I know and nothing can shake my faith in that. Stand on the Word of God. Get a scripture that really "grabs" you.

The scripture that grabbed me, might not grab you!

The scripture that grabs you, might not grab me!

Every once in a while someone will give me a real revelation on a scripture they have and I stand there and look at them blankly. I think, "Really?"

It doesn't make a bit of sense to me.

But...it does to them!

They believe it!

And that's all it takes!

6   And By His Stripes...

But He was wounded for our transgressions,
He was bruised for our iniquities;
The chastisement for our peace was upon Him,
And by His stripes we are healed. (Isaiah 53:5)

There is probably no scripture on which more people have stood to receive their healing than the above, and yet all over the world it is also controversial!

Does that mean our healing takes place before we receive it, or does it mean that the provision is there for us *to be* a recipient?

My personal feelings are that the provision is there just as it is for salvation, but you are not saved until you are saved, and you are not healed until you are healed!

BUT...every once in a while I hear a testimony that shows me both sides are right, and if you can receive and maintain your healing through quoting that scripture, I'm with you all the way!

We were in Denmark and the host who drove us to and from the meetings had experienced a miraculous healing from Myasthinia Gravis. He was as healthy as anyone you've ever seen and ran all the time, keeping up with the hectic schedule we maintained. He gave us a copy of the testimony as he had experienced it and written it with a remark, "Please use this in any way you want to in order to help someone else!"

I was so impressed that I decided to share it with you. I was going to edit it, but felt his Danish ability to speak English was so interesting that my final decision was not to touch it. I hope you can feel in it what I felt in it.

The History of a Miracle-Bicycle
or
The Grace of God in November 1987
or
'Give, and you shall receive'.

This experience happened in November 1987 and is true and pure facts as confirmed by my wife Ruth and by my and your brother in Christ Ove Stage, the father of the little girl.

Some background information is necessary:

For many years, 1968-78, I had been partially lame (called: Myasthenia Gravis), and I was unable to dress myself, comb my hair, walk distances, do bicycling, swimming, drive car etc. in spite of much medicine, and my eyes had double-eyesight because my right eye could not move.

We: my faithful wife Ruth, 41 and nurse, and our daughters of 16 and 12 live in a Copenhagen suburb, Denmark. I am 46, a computer programmer. I enjoyed a very good health until 1968, when the paralysis suddenly seized every muscle in my body, and I had only 20 percent strength left.

Through the 1970-ties there were several crises, and I spent 9 days in respirator because I could not breathe. I have received the best treatments doctors can give and our fine Danish social system has been a great help to me.

However, the severe invalidating lameness remained and life-threatening crises came repeatedly.

Since 1978 God has healed me in a continuous process through the complete works of Jesus, who conquered the powers of the devil, and through forgiveness of our sins restored spiritual life in God, salvation and healing, for mankind.

Gradually my muscles regained former strength, and after many years suffering I became able to do without medicine, to dress myself, comb my hair, walk trips of 6 miles, drive our car, and live a 'normal' life. My eyes are completely healed and I use no glasses. There is still some weakness in my fingers. The doctors are happy with me too, they have no medical explanation to my healing.

All glory to God. I thank Him now and for ever.

However — when driving bicycle, swimming, playing the piano — which I did with great pleasure until 1968 — I felt that my body was still too weak for that.

Here in Denmark where cars and petrol are expensive due to high taxes, people do a lot of bicycling. Every Dane above 3 years owns a cycle which is used for transport up to 5 miles: to and from school, suburban train stations, work, fetching food-stuff in store etc.

I often tried driving our daughter Karoline's old 'children-size' bicycle where I could reach the ground with both feet sitting on the small seat. Karoline has now a 14-year-old-sized bicycle, and her old 6-year-size is seldom used. But I could not drive and move the pedals without losing my balance and tumbling. I felt the seat was far too small and that my back was too weak for the complicated work of keeping the balance.

In a talk after the prayer-meeting in our home on Tuesday October 27 in our prayer-group I learned that the 6-year old daughter of one of the families was in need of another bicycle. We decided to give her Karoline's old cycle, which was worn but well functioning.

But the cycle would not fit into the luggage room of their car, so we promised to bring them the cycle a few days later.

Rolling the cycle back to our house through the garden I — as often before — tried to drive it — the seat was still very small and I stepped forward with both feet on the ground, trying to move the pedals.

WOW — one rotation of the pedals — then another rotation. Praise, God, I was driving again after 19 years....

Two days later we had a two-mile bicycle trip to our urban center. I had to be very careful about stones and bumps and turning left and right and many stared at me driving that small bicycle.

I had some pain in my behind because of the little seat, and the muscles around the knees were hurting and like jelly because they had not been used that way for 19 years.

Sunday November 1, at the morning service in the church, we met the family again. We told them that we would bring them the "miracle-bicycle" in a few weeks, when I would feel strong enough to drive one of my daughter's bigger bicycle.

They told us that the old cycle of their daughter had been stolen two days before and they were going to buy another one for her as she used it every day to school. We promised to bring the bicycle "as soon as possible·"

Monday November 2, I felt bad about the bicycle, because I was making the little girl wait.

I put it into our car and brought it to them. The daughter was very happy; her own cycle had been found destroyed.

Coming home that night I immediately took the big cycle of one of our daughters — and — all thanks to God — I was able to drive it...for the first time....

Wednesday November 4, I was driving my wife's bicycle. The seat is still "small", but WHAT a feeling driving again after 19 years, feeling the wind blowing because of the speed.

This miracle happened in just a week's time, and it will change our daily routines, just the same way it happened when God enabled me to drive car again, which happened two years ago. Jesus pro-

vided complete salvation and healing giving His life
for me at Calvary — I have received it gradually bit-
by-bit.

Many dear brothers and sisters have stood by
my side in prayers. You know, sometimes there is a
fight against evil powers. But Praise God, through
His Holy Spirit He has given His power, love and
anointing to men and women who committed themselves to be like Jesus and follow Him, think like
Him, believe like Him, preach like Him, pray like
Him, walking in the Spirit and not in the flesh.

I am thankful to them too — just like the
people of Malta, when the apostle Paul had stranded
on their island and brought to them the grace and
miracles of God.

Can you imagine our joy?

We are all so encouraged and praising God because of Jesus, 'by His stripes I am healed'

October 1989:

This testimony was written November '87 just
one week after it happened.

Since April '88 I drive bicycle to and from
work, a little more than 5 miles, when it is not rain-
ing or snowing.

At the sports event in the bank where I am
working I walk 10 km., 9 miles,. in 1 hour 16 min.

In Sept. '88 my correspondence with social au-
thorities was finished. The social pension was finally withdrawn, and we returned the 'handicapped
car' and bought our own.

It is fantastic to compare the doctor's documents from the 1970-ties with the new documents.

All Glory and Praise to Jesus!

-s- Carl Michael Pahus

Probably the thing that made me want to read this when he squeezed it into my hand was what his wife said, "Suddenly one day words came alive to me. I don't know the whole scripture, I only know that in one moment the words 'And by His stripes we are healed' became a reality!"

May they become a reality to you, too!

7 To Forgive Is To Receive To Forget Is To Maintain

For if ye forgive men their trespasses, your heavenly Father will also forgive you: But if ye forgive not men their trespasses, neither will your Father forgive your trespasses (Matthew 6:14-15 KJV).

As I meditated on writing this chapter on forgiveness, I reflected, "This has been taught many times! What new taste or new flavor can I give to it to make people realize how important forgiveness really is in receiving and maintaining a healing."

The most miserable unhappy people in the world are those who have unforgiveness in their hearts because eventually this leads to bitterness, resentment, hate, anger and many other attitudes which do not belong in a Christian's life. As I was reading through the Bible contemplating what I was going to say, the following verses really spoke to me concerning why some people have difficulty receiving a healing.

Come unto me, all ye that labour and are heavy laden, and I will give you rest. Take my yoke upon you, and learn of me; for I am meek and lowly in heart: and ye shall find rest unto your souls. For my yoke is easy, and my burden is light (Matthew 11:28-30 KJV).

As I read that particular scripture, suddenly it was as if God was saying, "People who don't give away their sickness to Me have difficulty being healed because they have not rid themselves of something that could often cause the sickness in their body."

This was brought to me very vividly at a recent Healing Explosion when Charles and I called the cancer victims to come up. A lady who had terminal cancer was in a wheelchair, and her healing card was laying on the top of a tray across the wheelchair.

Physically, she was in a pathetic condition but as I glanced at the card I saw she was in a worse condition spiritually. She had written: "I need to be healed of:

Lust
Bitterness
Resentment
Hate
Anger
Jealousy
Self-pity
Selfishness
Envy"
The list was endless!

The shock I experienced was unimaginable when I read all of the things for which she was asking to be healed! These are not things you can be healed of — these are things you have to get rid of yourself. As I laid hands on her I wondered how God could or would possibly heal someone who had all of these bad attitudes in their heart.

Her face showed it! The sound of her voice showed it! The look in her eyes showed it! It was obvious she hated the entire world! I even wondered if she didn't hate God because she blamed Him for the cancer which had put her in a wheelchair.

We saw no sign of healing whatsoever!

It often times amazes both of us when people come forward for healing, how they can expect to receive God's best when they are not willing to give Him their best.

To receive healing we need to forgive.

To maintain healing we need to forget.

How can you find rest for your soul when you have bitterness, hatred and anger in your heart? Jesus said His yoke was easy and His burden was light. When He says, *"Come unto me, all you who labor and are heavy laden, and I will give you rest,"* I believe that includes sickness as much as anything else. A prime requisite for healing is to get rid of any bad attitudes you may have.

People with unforgiveness in their hearts are for the most part people who are always determined to have their way. With God it's a question of His way and not your way.

His promises are so fantastic I don't know how

anybody would want to refuse the guarantee He
gives when He says, if you're heavy laden, come to
Him because His burden is light!

*A good man out of the good treasure of the
heart bringeth forth good things: and an evil man
out of the evil treasure bringeth forth evil things*
(Matthew 12:35 KJV).

When evil things come out of a person's mouth,
it is obvious there is bitterness, hate, anger and resentment inside of their heart.

The greatest example of this is when Jesus
hung on the cross! After the shame and torture Jesus
went through when He was crucified, He forgave
them!

The story of Stephen as told in the book of Acts
is another example of ultimate forgiveness!

Your faith really is put into full play when
someone comes against you, but read the rest of the
verses and see what Stephen did.

*And they stoned Stephen, calling upon God,
and saying, Lord Jesus, receive my spirit. And he
kneeled down, and cried with a loud voice, Lord, lay
not this sin to their charge* (Acts 7:59-60 KJV).

In other words what he really said was, "I forgive them. I do not care what they did to me, I forgive them." For this reason Stephen is recorded in
the Bible. If he had not forgiven them, he would
never have appeared in the Word of God.

We need to remember instances like this because when our spouse or our children do us wrong,
it's easy to get resentment against them. Unfortunately, resentment is like yeast. The more it sits, the

bigger it gets and it doesn't take long to be totally out of control!

I remember when I was a little child, probably 7 or 8 years old, we were at my grandparents' farm for the summer. Grandma had made some special homemade bread and put it in a little "warming" oven to raise. Then she and Grandpa left to pick peaches on a neighboring farm. When she left, she told us to be sure and watch the dough and when it got about one inch above the pan, we were to take it out and put it in the oven so the bread would bake by the time they got home for lunch.

We decided to ride the plow horses instead! My uncle put the bridle on and we were really having a wonderful time when suddenly we saw the wagon coming up the road with Grandma and Grandpa in it and we realized that the bread was still in the warming oven!

We jumped off the horses real quick — our young uncle who was the same age as we were, ran the horses to the barn, and then came running after us! When we got in the kitchen, I wish you could have seen that stove and warming oven! The dough was oozing all over the place and if I ever saw anything in my life that was out of control it was the bread we were supposed to be having for lunch! It had run out of the warming oven, down the side of the oven, over the floor and it looked like a river of "goo!"

Needless to say my uncle got a good whipping from his father, but because grandchildren have a special place in grandparents' hearts, nothing happened to my sister and me except we volunteered never to do it again, after we cleaned up the mess.

Often times when I think about unforgiveness I remember the bread with the yeast in it which kept getting bigger and bigger until it got totally out of control.

Unforgiveness is exactly the same way. It can start off with a minute little thing, and then as we let it fester in our mind and in our heart and in our spirit, unforgiveness can become something so big that it gets totally out of control.

Jesus forgave His disciples!

In fact, Jesus forgave you while you were still sinning.

Jesus said (Matthew 6:15), Your Father will not forgive you unless you forgive others. That's a serious promise, but Oh, the blessings when we forgive AND GOD FORGIVES!

Don't go on a guilt-trip, but take a close look at your life if you're not receiving healing, and see if there is some area that needs to be taken care of.

Ask the Holy Spirit to reveal anything to you which might be blocking your healing. He knows the answer!

8   Do You Want To?

By Charles

God wants us to trust Him and obey Him more than anything else. The worst sin against God is unbelief because when we have it, we are saying, "God, I really don't trust you."

Now when He rose early on the first day of the week, He appeared first to Mary Magdalene, out of whom He had cast seven demons.

She went and told those who had been with Him, as they mourned and wept.

And when they heard that He was alive and had been seen by her, THEY DID NOT BELIEVE.

After that, He appeared in another form to two of them as they walked and went into the country.

And they went and told it to the rest, BUT THEY DID NOT BELIEVE THEM EITHER.

(Mark 16:9-12)

Why not believe Him, trust Him, and then do what He wants us to do.

Is that easier said than done? Perhaps the reason God let's us grow in our trust is that if we could "magically" get anything we wanted, we would want the things God has made for us, instead of the God who made these things.

My favorite scripture is Philippians 2:13 quoted from The Living Bible, *"For God is at work within you, helping you want to obey him, and then helping you do what he wants."*

Once I really WANTED to please God instead of Charles, it became much easier to trust and obey Him. God shined His great light into the recesses of my heart and soul, then showed me the "little" things which were not pleasing Him, and then I discovered they were not pleasing me either.

When God spoke to me saying, "Go into My word, and listen to no man, and let ME tell you what I want you to know," I read thousands of hours in the Bible, seeking God and Jesus and what they wanted of me, and not what I wanted of them. That totally changed my life, and I began to learn the secret of obedience.

In relation to how to receive and maintain our healing, certain scriptures began to point out secrets of what trusting and obeying God really meant. I found myself short over and over again, but each time God showed me something I wasn't doing to please Him, or things I was doing which didn't please Him, I instantly started correcting my course. That was what I discovered pleased God — correcting myself to get into alignment with what pleased Him.

I once remarked from the depth of my heart, "God and Jesus, I would rather die than to do anything which is not pleasing to you, or to not do any-thing you want." I meant that, and have persistently lived up to the very intent of that thought, that promise. God didn't do it all at once, and is still oc-casionally showing me something else in my inner life which isn't up to the perfection He desires (for our benefit), but each time, I very quickly, methodi-cally, correct the course of my life or thinking.

It is the thought-life that pollutes. For from within, out of men's hearts, come evil thoughts of lust, theft, murder, adultery, wanting what belongs to others, wickedness, deceit, lewdness, envy, slan-der, pride, and all other folly. All these vile things come from within; they are what pollute you and make you unfit for God (Mark 7:20-23 TLB).

From this and other "conversation thoughts" between God and me, I realized that attitudes, our inner thoughts which were not pleasing to God and Jesus, were the heart of all my problems in pleasing Them.

Herein lies much of our difficulty in trusting and obeying God to receive or maintain our heal-ings.

I used to wonder why Jesus said it was worse to hate your brother than to murder. Then I realized you would not murder if you did not first hate. In-side us, in our thought-life, in our attitudes, our in-tentions, our choice of pleasing God or ourselves, can be the root of our sicknesses and diseases.

So I want men everywhere to pray with holy hands lifted up to God, free from sin and anger and resentment (I Timothy 2:8 TLB).

Notice the many instructions from the Holy Spirit in the following scriptures, and how very simple they are. I love Frances' summation of pleasing God: "Do what God tells you to do and stop doing what He tells you not to do!" In the books of Galatians, Ephesians, Philippians, Colossians, and on through the various letters in the New Testament, we find plenty of instructions about how to live for Jesus, and health and healing naturally follow living His way.

Here are just a few samples of instructions which are in the New Testament:

Let me say this, then, speaking for the Lord: Live no longer as the unsaved do, for they are blinded and confused. Their closed hearts are full of darkness; they are far away from the life of God because they have shut their minds against him, and they cannot understand his ways. They don't care anymore about right and wrong and have given themselves over to impure ways. They stop at nothing, being driven by their evil minds and reckless lusts.

"But that isn't the way Christ taught you! If you have really heard his voice and learned from him the truths concerning himself, then throw off your old evil nature—the old you that was a partner in your evil ways—rotten through and through, full of lust and sham.

Now your attitudes and thoughts must all be constantly changing for the better. Yes, you must be a new and different person, holy and good. Clothe yourself with this new nature.

Stop lying to each other; tell the truth, for we are parts of each other and when we lie to each other we are hurting ourselves. If you are angry, don't sin by nursing your grudge. Don't let the sun go down with you still angry—get over it quickly; for when you are angry you give a mighty foothold to the devil.

If anyone is stealing he must stop it and begin using those hands of his for honest work so he can give to others in need. Don't use bad language. Say only what is good and helpful to those you are talking to, and what will give them a blessing.

Don't cause the Holy Spirit sorrow by the way you live. Remember, he is the one who marks you to be present on that day when salvation from sin will be complete.

Stop being mean, bad-tempered and angry. Quarreling, harsh words, and dislike of others should have no place in your lives. Instead, be kind to each other, tender-hearted, forgiving one another, just as God has forgiven you because you belong to Christ (Ephesians 4:17-32 TLB).

Let there be no sex sin, impurity or greed among you. Let no one be able to accuse you of any such things. Dirty stories, foul talk and coarse jokes—these are not for you. Instead, remind each other of God's goodness and be thankful.

You can be sure of this: The kingdom of Christ and of God will never belong to anyone who is impure or greedy, for a greedy person is really an idol worshiper—he loves and worships the good things of this life more than God. Don't be fooled by those

who try to excuse these sins, for the terrible wrath of
God is upon all those who do them (Ephesians 5:3-6
TLB).

I began to look closely at my life and attitudes
to see if I really was pleasing God. He made it very
plain in some of these areas that I could improve
considerably.

If we really examine our attitudes and habits,
we can discover at least some of the reasons we do
not receive our healings, or we lose them once we
have received them.

It was my old evil nature which constantly
kept me from the abundant life Jesus wanted me to
have, and until I cried out from my heart to God,
"Take all of my life and make me spiritually what
you want me to be," I couldn't overcome these attitudes that constantly pulled me into myself, my
old carnal nature. I was not obeying all of God's
laws, and I knew it.

If someone did me wrong, I would "sort of" get
mad at them. I didn't hesitate to make cutting remarks (with nice words), always trying to look good
in the eyes of others, but hurting those who were
near me. I wasn't really that bad all the time, but
just enough of the time to know I wasn't pleasing
God.

I found myself violating many of these simple
principles which are in the verses quoted above. I
didn't want to do them, but I did anyway.

What was I really doing? I was disobeying
what God commanded quoted above in Ephesians,
so what effect did that have on my receiving and

maintaining a healing? God's promises proved true, mostly on the bad side, but at least not living in the abundance Jesus desired for my life, and yours.

What can we do to put ourselves in alignment with God's promises? "Do what God tells you to do, and stop doing what He tells you not to do."

In our book ANGELS ON ASSIGNMENT there is a mighty truth revealed which I want to repeat here for you which I believe will connect attitudes to sickness, obedience of God's laws to health, disobedience of God to sicknesses:

This is quoted from the chapter "My Visit to the Throne Room", pages 56 and 57:

"Another of the extremely interesting things God told me when I was with Him was about outer space. God spoke of the graveyards of stars in outer space. I talked to my wife about it, and she was as amazed as I was.

"There has been a lot of speculation about the empty spaces in heaven. He explained that the reason it appears that there are dark, empty spaces, is that the gravitational pull of stars inside of themselves is so strong that it bends their light rays back inside, so the stars go out and consequently they do not give out light rays any more. The black holes do not mean that there are no stars there, but simply that their light has gone out and they cannot be seen. The black holes are the graveyards of stars. God said that when our thoughts turn inward, we become just like the stars that are wandering in darkness. . ."

"He also reminded me that the earth is a wonderful place, because the whole earth is filled with

His glory! He let me see an increasing number of people turning to him. Not a people backing away, not a surrendering of the church, not a church heading underground, but a church triumphant!"

Satan turned inward in heaven and his glory and light went out because of wanting to please himself instead of pleasing God.

Satan came to earth to Eve and convinced her that if she would disobey God (turn inward and prize herself and her desires above God) she would gain. But when she turned inward, her light went out; she lost her soul and the wonderful, beautiful place on earth provided by God. I'm sure sickness entered into her body and the body of her family and descendants— including us.

When our desire to please ourselves instead of pleasing God turns us inward, sicknesses begin and poverty begins in our lives (not necessarily financial poverty, but poverty of other failures in our lives. Marriage for example. When we want to please ourselves, we are in constant combat with our spouse and family).

When we turn inward, we find that every negative attitude arises within us, and no longer can we be the light of the world, we cannot even reflect the light of Jesus.

Peter is a perfect example of this. He loved Jesus with all his heart, and gave up his fishing business to follow Jesus. But the carnal, self-nature in Peter turned him inward when it was either his life taken or that of Jesus. He protected himself, and let Jesus down when his Master needed him the most.

That was exactly what ruled my life as a carnal Christian.

But something happened to Peter and Charles when we both made an absolute, total commitment to Jesus and turned outward instead of inward: Tongues of fire came on Peter and burned out that fleshly, self-directed nature on the day of Pentecost; in 1968, I didn't see tongues of fire, but I'm quite sure that same thing happened to me when I cried out silently from the depth of my soul, "God, take all of my life and make me spiritually what You want me to be."

Abundant life started for me; God cleaned out my self-desires and turned them outward toward God and Jesus, and toward seeing what I could do to please Them instead of me.

My ulcers soon cleared; frequent constipation left; my hayfever left; tenseness which caused much discomfort left; a peace and joy flooded my soul night and day, year after year, and continues to this day. My anxiety left; my self-pity left; my anger left; my cutting remarks turned to ministering to others; fear of heart problems left; fear of lightning and fear of death left.

At the time of this writing, 22 years later, I am age 70 and in perfect health almost all the time, and my body is young and strong. My eyesight is clear; my ears hear normally; all of my body functions work perfectly.

Most of all, I can reflect the light of Jesus as I turn outward to minister to others through teaching, training others, through writing books which can change lives of people we never see. Through bringing salvation, the baptism with the Holy Spirit, ministering healing and deliverance, and making disciples for Jesus.

My hearty recommendation is: Turn outward and let the world see your light as the light of Jesus: this brings peace, joy, love, and all the other fruit of the Spirit; health, strength, prosperity in all ways.

If the stars can do it, you can do it too! If Charles and Frances can do it, you can do it too!

UNFORGIVENESS: Just after the Lord's prayer, Matthew 6:14,15 TLB: *Your heavenly Father will forgive you if you forgive those who sin against you; but if you refuse to forgive them, he will not forgive you.*

Can you see the strong words of God here? Could unforgiveness cause us even to miss heaven just through not forgiving someone?

What can this do for our health, or loss of it? We hear from doctors that arthritis is often caused by unforgiveness, bitterness, hate, envy, jealousy. The balance in our body systems begin to work against one another and our nerves begin to malfunction; apparently this causes "dry bones" as spoken of in the Bible. Dry bones, the marrow, means that the red blood cells are not being produced.

WORRY-ANXIETY: Jesus gave a rather long teaching on this in Matthew 6:19-24. I had just read an article on STRESS, and turned to this portion of scripture. Jesus identified the causes and effects, and gave the solutions in a few words. *So don't worry at all about having enough food and clothing.*

Why be like the heathen? For they take pride in all these things and are deeply concerned about them. But your heavenly Father already knows perfectly well that you need them, and he will give them to you if you give Him first place in your life and live as He wants you to.

So don't be anxious about tomorrow. God will take care of your tomorrow too. Live one day at a time (Matthew 6:31-34 TLB).

In the article I was reading, the author stated, "No living organism can exist continuously in a state of alarm." Stress seems to be somewhat the talk of the streets today. Article after article is written about coping with stress. Of course, the ideal is to avoid stress. We may not be able to avoid it, but we certainly can do a lot about controlling its cause through these attitude eruptions and hanging on to the attitudes (letting the sun go down while we are still angry).

If you really want to maintain your diseases, sicknesses, and pains, mix the following ingredients and you will succeed in perpetual ailments and sicknesses:

Worry	Self pity
Anxiety	Wrong inclinations
Fear	Criticism
Hate	Complaining
Resentment	Bitterness
Jealousy	Martyr complex
Imaginations and strong holds	
Suspicion	Guilt
Negative attitudes and expressions	

At the very root of all these negative attitudes lies SELF. Satan wanted to be like God (idolatry, selfishness) and he rebelled against God's laws. Resistance against our natural health laws will cause a heavy mixture of the above attitudes. The only two sins which will take us out from under the covering of the blood of Jesus once we are born-again are idolatry and rebellion. The biggest idol we can have is ourselves — putting "self" above God. When we idolize ourself and our desires above the desires and ways of God, we are rebelling against God's laws.

It has been scientifically proven that negative attitudes are energy forces which are destructive. Positive attitudes are energy forces which are constructive, including our health and peace. If there are questions about this, just ask any doctor.

What are the antidotes for such sicknesses, diseases, stress, and other negative effects on our minds, bodies, and souls?

Just to be sure of the meaning of the word "antidote", I looked in the dictionary and found some interesting facts:

ANTIDOTE: A remedy to counteract the effects of poison, or of anything noxious taken into the system. Anything tending to counteract an evil; as, an antidote for poverty.

To provide an antidote for, as a disease or condition.

Changing from bad to good attitudes means changing from disobedience of God's conditions (curses and sickness) to obedience of His laws (blessings and health).

Do you want to get rid of a bad attitude?

First, you have to admit you have one...

There are two forces always competing for our desires: The old evil nature that gives us the bad attitudes, and wrong thinking and selfish motives; and the Holy Spirit who tells us what to do, thereby opening our pathways into blessings and health.

Galatians 5:16-18 (TLB): *I advise you to obey only the Holy Spirit's instructions. He will tell you where to go and what to do, and then you won't always be doing the wrong things your evil nature wants you to. For we naturally love to do evil things that are just the opposite from the things that the Holy Spirit tells us to do; and the good things we want to do when the Spirit has his way with us are just the opposite of our natural desires. These two forces within us are constantly fighting each other to win control over us, and our wishes are never free from their pressures. When you are guided by the Holy Spirit you need no longer force yourself to obey Jewish laws.*

Galatians 5:22-23 (TLB): *But when the Holy Spirit controls our lives he will produce this kind of fruit in us: love, joy, peace, patience, kindness, goodness, faithfulness, gentleness, and self-control; and here there is no conflict with Jewish laws.*

Attitudes can eat us up like a cancer that just keeps eating, and eating, and eating until we destroy ourselves. It is not the devil doing this, although he is in there trying all the time to convince us we have a right to these attitudes; it is our own choosing, and we can break the habits and release these bad germs of sickness. How? Give them to Jesus, and start trying to please Him with every thought, intent, and attitude. Practice good attitudes on others; try smiling cheerfully at the next 100 people you meet. You will discover that most of them will smile back.

Try keeping a bad disposition as you meet the next 100 people and you will feel that the whole world is mad at you. As a child, I was told that it takes 13 times more energy to frown than to smile. I chose at that early age to always smile, and my life has been full of joy — and friends.

We must concentrate and discipline ourselves to keep from practicing negative words and forces in our lives, and as we do that, replace them with good and healthy words and attitudes.

Attitudes are not the only things which keep us from being healed or keeping our healings.

Many hygiene habits and actions can contribute to our healing and health, along with common sense and normal knowledge. We actually can bring health or sickness into our bodies and minds by our own choices, but generally without knowing we are doing such things. Think about some of the following hints for health:

1. Drink eight glasses of water daily. God invented water and nobody has improved upon it. I often say that to waitresses when they ask what we would like to drink. But generally this is followed by, "Do you know Jesus as your Savior?" We have led many people to Jesus in just that simple way.

Winning someone to Jesus brings an inner joy that nothing else will, and you can be sure it delights God and Christ Jesus, and even the angels of Heaven rejoice. Think what that kind of obedience does for your system.

2. "The joy of the Lord is our strength." Try perpetually living with joy in your heart and watch your health improve. That isn't a cure-all, but it sure beats sadness which draws your strength from you.

Marilyn Hickey once remarked to us, "The joy of the Lord is your strength, because you always project joy into other people." We realize that there are times of trials and difficult unpleasing situations, but they don't need to remove your joy. Consider this motto: The joy of the Lord is my strength; the lack of joy in the Lord drains my strength.

3. *"A merry heart doeth good like a medicine"* (Prov. 17:22). It does! Try looking into your mirror and laughing for a few minutes early in the morning. It works wonders. Try looking up to God with a big smile and sing a praise song to Him in your Spirit language; then see how quickly bad attitudes leave.

Luke 11:36 (TLB): *If you are filled with light within, with no dark corners, then your face will be radiant too, as though a floodlight is beamed upon you.*

If we really believe the joy of the Lord is our strength; that a merry heart doeth good like a medicine; that Jesus is the answer to every problem in life; that Jesus actually saved us and brought us the opportunity to have life abundantly; then our faces should show this wherever we go, day and night, in trouble or in pleasant times, in sickness and in health. Our faces were made to reflect God's light, but we must choose our own disposition and reflection. It can affect our health.

4. Keep our bodies clean, including our teeth. It shocks me when I see executive businessmen leave a restroom without washing their hands. A witness is often destroyed when our breath is not fresh; but our teeth also lose their health. Body odor is destructive to friendship and success, and affects our health adversely.

We once had a young accountant working in our firm who really was good at his job. But every time I was near him, I could hardly stand the odor. We are very reluctant to tell someone of a problem like this, but one day I knew I had to help him. I very lovingly told him about it. He thanked me sincerely. It was only a short time until he was working as an executive with an increase of at least three times his salary. Besides that, the pores of our skin are for breathing and should be kept clean and open for elimination of body poisons.

5. We know a lady who decided to murder her husband. She put just a little poison in his food every morning until he died. She is still in prison after many, many years. Praise God, she found Jesus and is a dynamic witness in the jail. I was thinking about this in relation to our food intake. If we knew we would die within thirty days if we took a certain amount of poison daily, but about the middle of that time we were cramping and violently sick, could we cry out to God, "God heal me" and get results if we

still planned to take poison the next day? Of course not.

In a similar manner, we put foods and drinks into our systems which are actually as destructive as poisons; but maybe not as fast working. Think about some of these: Alcohol, tobacco, drugs, caffeine, sugar, pork, too many greasy fast foods. Then think of what you have been taught: Plenty of fresh water, lots of fresh vegetables, the right kinds of meats, fruits, etc.

Common sense and a normal health guide book can go a long way in keeping us in health, if we will obey the laws God gave us. God's "health food" book is Leviticus and in this we can find a guide to healthy foods.

But what do most of us do? We go right on taking our little bit of poison every day in the form of food and drinks which we know will destroy us.

Do you not know that you are the temple of God and that the Spirit of God dwells in you? If anyone defiles the temple of God, God will destroy him. For the temple of God is holy, which temple you are (I Corinthians 3:16,17).

It is senseless for you to work so hard from early morning until late at night, fearing you will starve to death; for God wants His loved ones to get their proper rest (Psalm 127:2 TLB).

Our immune system is designed to resist diseases. If it is weakened or destroyed, we are subjected to every disease in the world. If we deliberately, or unknowingly, destroy our resistance to diseases by our habits and attitudes, we are inviting sicknesses into our bodies.

The more time we meditate in the Bible, the more we find a closeness to the one who took all of our sicknesses on His body, and the nearer we get to divine health. Frances and I have not quite attained divine health, but we certainly recover more quickly when we do catch some kind of a sickness.

Our favorite suggestion in reading the Bible is, "Father, what can I do to please you; not what you can do to please me." This opens great highways into abundant living, if we will listen and obey what God tells us to do!

Obedience is the foundation to serving God, and obedience because we want to is the route to easy obedience. I serve Frances in everything I can because I want to! If I did it because I had to, it would be drudgery. I choose the pleasant route to pleasing her, and it is wonderful! It also produces health because I always maintain joy in doing it, peace and happiness in doing it, and she also receives that same benefit. Frances also follows that same course of wanting to please me.

We both know that Jesus lives in us, so whatever we do or don't do to one another, we are doing it to Jesus. When we love each other and serve each other, we are pleasing the Jesus who lives in us. If we chose to complain, say wrong things, have wrong attitudes toward each other, we would have to look up to Jesus, and say, "That goes for you, too!"

Then He will answer them, saying, 'Assuredly, I say to you, inasmuch as you did not do it to one of the least of these, you did not do it to Me' (Matthew

25:45).

Jesus is talking: *Why do you call me, "Lord, Lord," but do not do what I say? Everyone who comes to me and listens to my words and obeys is like a man building a house. He digs deep and lays his foundation on rock. The floods come, and the water tries to wash the house away. But the flood cannot move the house, because the house was built well. But the one who hears my words and does not obey is like a man who builds his house on the ground without a foundation. When the floods come, the house quickly falls down. And that house is completely destroyed"* (Luke 6:46-49 EB).

The Bible tells us that if we give, we will receive. Jesus projected Himself into us to do the things He did, and even greater things. What happens if we give healing to others? We put ourselves in line for healing in our own bodies. If you smile at others, what do you get in return? A smile.

We know that continually ministering healing to others brings health to our own bodies. When the energy of God's Holy Spirit continues to flow through us, certainly that energy which heals others heals our own bodies.

If we really want to receive and maintain healing and health, we should realize that what God and Jesus say is an absolute truth. It cannot fail. All of God's words and the words spoken by Jesus are for our enjoyment and benefit. God wants us healthy, wealthy, and wise.

If we will study the suggestions described in this chapter, and in this book, we can discover how all that we are in health and happiness is found in the Bible, and we can attain everything God has designed for us. Even our bodies and minds were designed to be healthy. Cut your finger, and healing flows quickly to the injury and ministers healing.

Alex Schneider, a very close friend, made this comment about us, and we want to pass it on to you for your own application and health: He said, "I've seen you in adverse situations but your faith is so pure and simple that it doesn't affect your joy. Your assurance in God and Jesus perpetuates your outflowing joy, not only in yourselves, but outwardly to others." This is attainable by all of God's children, and will bless all who trust and obey God completely.

A minister friend developed a very highly successful church, along with schools, programs, and many excellent works beyond just his church activities. Then came strife, followed by tremendous stress as he tried to meet the demands of those who began to oppose him.

We met him sometime later and he said the doctor had diagnosed a serious heart problem. It was severe and genuinely a bad heart condition. The next time we saw him, he had also been diagnosed as having cancer. Life seemed to be coming to an end.

A solution came to the stressful situation, he moved to an entirely different environment and out of the stressful atmosphere. We saw him a year or so later and he looked wonderfully healthy. When we inquired, "What happened to you?" he said once he was out from under the stress, his health began to improve, and the doctor had diagnosed him as having neither cancer or heart problems. Hallelujah!

What had happened? God and his body wanted him to be healthy and when he met God's conditions, God's laws of health worked wonders for him!

There is no end, no limit, no height, nor depth, nor length to the masses of promises God placed in His word just for us, but we must seek Him, seek to please Him, and obey every one of His laws if we want to receive and maintain health.

Finally: *Beloved, I pray that you may prosper in all things and be in health, just as your soul prospers* (3 John: 2).

How can we attain that promise of God? If we bring our soul into alignment with those words, it will prosper. Then the other promises will follow — we may prosper in all things and be in health."

When any disease strikes us, the doctor will seek the underlying cause, and then prescribe treatment. If you have a boil on your body, treating the outside will have little or no effect, but if you remove the core, or cause, of the boil, then it will find health.

If we are having health problems, or failing to maintain our healings, we should seek the cause and cure. It is not always something we are doing in our attitudes or habits, but so very often that is the case.

Look for these and other causes:

The foods you eat, the liquids you drink.

The hours you rest, or don't rest. (Prayer meetings lasting past midnight are dangerous).

Your attitudes: good or bad.

Your habits: good or bad.

How much time do you spend reading your Bible, and when reading are you saying, "Father, what can I do to please you, and not what can you do to please me?"

Do you live to serve God's spiritual food to others, or are you thinking about yourself. Turn outward and let the light of Jesus shine; not inward where there is darkness.

Do you not only attend church regularly, but do you serve others physically, mentally, and spiritually?

Seek health (obedience to God's laws); not cures.

Seek God, not the things God made.

Forgive those who have hurt us by loving their souls, then we can love them.

WANT TO BE HEALTHY AND HAPPY! WANT TO DO IT GOD'S WAY!

Finally, brethren, whatever things are true, whatever things are noble, whatever things are just, whatever things are pure, whatever things are lovely, whatever things are of good report, if there is any virtue and if there is anything praiseworthy — meditate on these things. (Philippians 4:8,9).

I know how to be abased, and I know how to abound. Everywhere and in all things I have learned both to be full and to be hungry, both to abound and to suffer need. I CAN DO ALL THINGS THROUGH CHRIST WHO STRENGTHENS ME. (Philippians

4:12,13).

In all my life I never smoked any tobacco, drank any alcohol, took any drugs, but I did have a minor amount of bad attitudes.

God showed me something which I believe can help you in being delivered from habits or attitudes.

Peter loved Jesus, gave up his business to follow Him, and would do anything to please Jesus. Then came the testing time. Jesus told Peter that he would deny Him before the rooster crowed. Peter said he would rather die than do that, and Peter meant that with all his heart.

But a choice came when Peter realized that if the ones persecuting Jesus knew that he was with Jesus, they would destroy him also. Knowing this, Peter had a choice, and he chose to please Peter (protect his own life rather than that of Jesus), so he denied and even cursed Jesus.

Then came the day of Pentecost when two things happened to Peter. He was endued with power when the Holy Spirit came upon him, and he spoke with other tongues — the baptism with the Holy Spirit. The other thing which happened was that tongues like as of fire came on Peter. This fire was the cleansing, purifying, purging fire of God's Holy Spirit, and just as the flesh of animals was burned to dead ashes as sin offerings in the Old Testament, so was the fleshly nature, the selfish nature of Peter, burned into nothingness.

Immediately, Peter rose up with boldness to proclaim Jesus, risking his very life, but no longer did Peter try to protect himself. What had happened? Peter now had Christ in Him, and it was no longer Peter who lived, but Jesus who lived in him.

Now Peter wanted to please Jesus instead of himself. He crucified his desires to please himself, and did what pleased Jesus.

Peter, who had loved his desires more than those of Jesus, now loved Jesus more than he loved Peter.

When that happened to me in 1968, I realized that when I had a bad attitude creep up on me, I tried to protect me, but the Holy Spirit reminded me that if I were dead to self, I no longer would try to please me. I had the power to reverse my attitudes and to please Jesus and His desires, rather than my own.

I believe we can always get rid of any habits or attitudes which are not pleasing to God and Christ Jesus if we love to please Jesus more than to please our own desires by continuing the bad habits and attitudes.

9   I Will Praise Him!

How I praise God for all the healings He has given me! Charles often says I have more new parts than original parts!

I praise Him for the new thyroid He gave me the day I was saved!

I praise Him for the new adrenal glands He gave me the day I was saved which brought about my healing from Addison's disease immediately!

I praise Him for the new heart He gave me in 1974!

I praise Him for the new pancreas He gave me in 1985 when He healed me of diabetes!

I praise Him for the entire new blood system He inserted into my body in 1988!

I praise Him for the protection He has given us as we have traveled all over the world!

And I will praise Him every day of my life!

Some of you are saying: "That's easy for you, because you have all of your prayers answered! I'd serve God like you do if He would just heal me!"

As I am writing this book, an interesting situation has occurred!

Eighteen years ago I fell down two little steps in the dark. No problem, and it never hurt, but twelve years after that, we were in Bogota, Colombia. We had a glorious service and saw more than 100 people come out of wheelchairs and off of crutches! What a day to remember...*but I left Colombia in a wheelchair!*

How I ever survived the trip from Colombia to Miami, I will never know! It was excruciating! We called our secretary and told her to make an appointment with an orthopedic doctor because my knee was swollen almost bigger than my head!

Prayer was the only thing that got me from Miami to Houston, and we went to the specialist directly from the airport where he removed more than a pint of water from my knee! That is extremely painful!

The knee continued to cause such agonizing pain that I couldn't stand, I couldn't sit, I couldn't lay down! After praying fervently and without ceasing, I finally had orthoscopic surgery on the knee.

The knee has given me a slight amount of pain most of the time, but about six months ago, it became acute! We have prayed, we have believed, we have done everything I have told you to do, but as of this writing, I am still walking bone on bone on my right knee. The cartilage is completely destroyed and in desperation, we have made an appointment to have a knee replacement done!

Either God will heal my knee and give me a

new one before you read this book, or I will have a replacement! The doctors have allowed me to continue our hectic schedule because I did not want to cancel any of our speaking dates, but they told me I would have to sit down to minister! God has been gracious, and the shot of cortisone they gave me was anointed (the physician is a Christian) and I have had a minimum amount of pain.

Audiences all over the nation have prayed for me in almost every service but the new knee hasn't come into being YET!

You may wonder why I'm telling you this! It is for a very special reason!

I have heard many people say, "If God would heal me, I would really be a witness for Him. I would really serve Him."

My last words to you in this book are, "I'll love God and serve God all the days of my life whether He heals me or not! It doesn't affect my love for Him nor my faith in Him and I will always believe that NOTHING IS IMPOSSIBLE WITH GOD!"

When (and if) the surgeon's knife makes the first cut into my flesh, I will still be witnessing about Him, His healing power, His majesty and His love!

And I will serve Him all the days of my life!